Healing Places

Healing Places

Wilbert M. Gesler

ROWMAN & LITTLEFIELD PUBLISHERS, INC.
Lanham • Boulder • New York • Oxford

ROWMAN & LITTLEFIELD PUBLISHERS, INC.

Published in the United States of America
by Rowman & Littlefield Publishers, Inc.
A Member of the Rowman & Littlefield Publishing Group
4501 Forbes Blvd., Suite 200, Lanham, Maryland 20706
www.rowmanlittlefield.com

PO Box 317, Oxford OX2 9RU, United Kingdom

British Library Cataloguing in Publication Information Available

Library of Congress Cataloging-in-Publication Data
Gesler, Wilbert M., 1941–
   Healing places / Wilbert M. Gesler.
      p. cm.
Includes bibliographical references and index.
   ISBN 0-7425-1955-4 (cloth : alk. paper) — ISBN 0-7425-1956-2 (paper : alk. paper)
   1. Hospital architecture. 2. Healing. 3. Medical geography. 4. Health resorts. 5.
Environment health. I. Title.
   RA967 .G475 2003
   613'.122—dc21

                                                                2002155384

Printed in the United States of America

♾™ The paper used in this publication meets the minimum requirements of
American National Standard for Information Sciences—Permanence of Paper for
Printed Library Materials, ANSI/NISO Z39.48-1992.

To my parents: Frances, George,
Margaret, Jane, Bob, and Elisabeth

Contents

Acknowledgments

My most sincere thanks go to several people who encouraged me to pursue therapeutic landscape or healing place ideas: Karen Reeds was the first to urge me to write a book; Robin Kearns and Alison Williams have been strong supporters of these healing concepts; Sarah Curtis and Brian Blundell introduced the notion of hospital design; Morag Bell kept the hospital design idea alive and added a critical perspective; several anonymous reviewers shaped the journal articles and book chapters on which much of the book is based; and Brenda Hadenfeldt, my editor at Rowman & Littlefield, enthusiastically moved the book along to publication. Thank you all.

CHAPTER ONE

⁂

Introduction

Healing and place are inseparable. Everyone can think of a specific place where they would like to be while being treated for or recuperating from a serious illness. For some it might be home where mother or some other relative or friend will take care of them; for others it might be a tropical island, a cabin in the mountains, even a hospital or hospice where the staff are known to be caring. Many people mention specific places they think of as healing places: Hot Springs, Arkansas; Asheville, North Carolina; Denali Park, Alaska; the Mayo Clinic, Minnesota; and many, many others.

There is a great deal of current interest in creating therapeutic environments in places such as hospitals (Gesler, Bell, and Curtis 2002). Many people do not feel at all comfortable in a hospital and hardly think of it as a healing place. However, a variety of people, including architects, hospital management, staff, and patients, believe that changes can be made in a hospital to provide a place that is conducive to physical, mental, spiritual, emotional, and social healing. Since at least the time of Florence Nightingale it has been recognized that providing fresh air, adequate lighting, good accommodation for staff, and other amenities were aids to the healing process (Nightingale 1863). Many hospitals and clinics in recent years have attempted to improve their environments by introducing, as examples, trees onto their grounds, painting walls in pastel

1

colors, or using *feng shui* in building design (Purvis 2001). It is, however, very difficult to evaluate the effect of introducing a feature like artwork in a hospital (Miles 1997).

It is clear that people associate places with healing. But if asked *why* places heal, their answers are not so readily forthcoming. "Nature heals" is the most common response. Some people mention the importance of social support and good doctor/patient communication. But most of us don't really think very much about these things; what specifically makes for a healing environment is not always immediately apparent. Many people would look for the medical practices of different times and places as the best clue to their success. This, however, is not a book about advances in medical technology. Rather, taking a humanistic approach, it looks for a variety of other, often more subtle clues as to why people think that certain places successfully heal.

One way to look for ideas about healing places would be to study a modern place such as a popular mineral spring or well-known hospital. I believe, however, that we can learn a great deal from looking at what has happened in the past. Then we can apply what has been learned to evaluate places that are intended to provide healing today. In this introductory chapter the goal is to answer the question of why some places achieved lasting reputations for healing or what I choose to call a healing sense of place. The logic of the argument is as follows. First, important aspects of the concept of healing are addressed: these include (1) its multidimensional character (physical, mental, spiritual, emotional, and social); (2) wholeness, connectedness, or integration; (3) healing from within; (4) an ongoing process with meaning in one's everyday life; and (5) healing as a humanistic approach. This last theme leads into a discussion of the idea from cultural geography (which is largely a humanistic subdiscipline) of sense of place and, in particular, a *healing sense of place*. Then the claim is made that there are four "environments" that contribute to a healing sense of place: natural, built, symbolic, and social. The ideas that lie behind this claim are not new, but are supported by research in the social sciences, medicine, and public health; the bulk of this chapter provides details of that research. The last step is to discuss how three places were chosen to illustrate the ways in which the four environments helped them to achieve lasting reputations for healing.

The Healing Process

The first word in the title of this book, healing, is very difficult to define. So, rather than attempt a definition here, I will set out some of the attributes or themes connected with healing that recur in the literature. A commonly encountered idea is that healing is multidimensional; it includes physical or biological, mental, spiritual, emotional, and social elements (Landis 1997; Moyers 1993). That is, getting well is not limited to a physical cure. The mind also has to be put at rest, one's spiritual and emotional needs must be met, and healthy social relationships must be maintained. Dividing healing into its components in this way might appear to multiply the problems encountered in getting well. On the other hand, thinking in a more positive way, one's physical, mental, spiritual, emotional, and social resources can all be brought to bear in a synergistic manner on the process of healing. The following examples demonstrate the importance that people concerned with health have given to nonbiological aspects of healing. Barnard Lown (1983), a well-known cardiologist, found from decades of experience with his patients that psychological factors affected all aspects of illness. In the opinion of B. J. Landis (1997), who is a nurse, spirituality is the key to healing. In his discussions with medical practitioners on the subject of healing, journalist Bill Moyers (1993) found that they stressed the importance of social supports and being able to express one's feelings to alleviate emotional pain.

The word heal derives from an Old English word *haelon*, which means wholeness. The parallel ideas of wholeness, connectedness, and integration run through the literature on healing. Quinn (1997, ix) puts the theme this way: "People are not collections of parts that need to be fixed, but whole bodymindspirits." The idea is that healing is facilitated by integrating the physical, mental, spiritual, emotional, and social components of a patient's being. Each of these components affects the other. Probably the most studied link among all the possibilities is the one between the mind and the body; it is clear from many studies that each influences the other and, in fact, they are inseparable (Frank and Frank 1991; Mehl 1986). Although the mechanisms are not clearly understood, we know that the mind affects the autonomic, endocrine, and immune systems. Thus, for example, positive attitudes and emotions can affect the biochemistry of the body to facilitate healing (Rossi 1986). In particular, the science of psychoneuroimmunology has studied the "messages" sent between the mind and the body (Landis 1997). Some scientists play down the importance of these connections as being merely the "placebo response." However, in the opinion of Rossi (1986), the placebo response can be put to positive use. Perhaps the most famous case is that of Norman Cousins who used the power of his mind (e.g., laughter and positive thinking) to overcome a life-threatening illness and a badly damaged heart (Lown 1983).

Another pervasive theme is that healing must come from within, that everyone has the innate capacity to heal themselves, and that this capacity must somehow be mobilized (Lown 1983). Whereas most treatment in the formal health care system is administered either by practitioners or machines, the contention is that healing can only come when patients marshal their inner resources (Fox 1993). Simply put, patients must *want* to get well and can do so if they coordinate their thoughts, spirituality, emotions, and social support in an effort to get better. This is not to say that others, professional healers in particular, are not important. Indeed, they are, not as disinterested practitioners of medicine, but as people who help patients help themselves (Moyers 1993). There needs to be a synergy between patient and practitioner, each helping the other to bring the resources they possess to bear (Fox 1993).

Yet another theme is healing as an ongoing experience, which is part of one's daily life (Kritek 1997). What is particularly important for people is that their lived experience has meaning for them. Healing is therefore made easier if a proposed treatment is meaningful to a person in terms of their physical, mental, spiritual, emotional, and social needs. We know, for example, what people should do if they have diabetes or wish to prevent it (e.g., eat a proper diet, exercise, and take medications on a regular basis), but compliance is often made difficult because prescriptions may not make sense in the context of lived experience (e.g., one finds it very hard to resist eating rich foods at social gatherings, one is too tired to exercise at the end of a day of manual labor, or medicines are too costly). Ways have to be found to make diabetes prevention and treatment meaningful in terms of people's everyday practices.

The healing concept arises from a humanistic perspective on the delivery of health care; the humanistic approach is our final theme. This approach puts the patient at the center. Howard et al. (1977, 12) state that humanistic health care is "care that enhances the dignity and autonomy of patients and professionals alike." It includes such things as giving patients accurate information about their illness, exploring the meaning of sickness and hospitalization with patients, and allowing patients to express their feelings about their experiences (Fenton 1997). Humanistic practitioners treat people as if they were unique and have inherent worth, strive to achieve wholeness (physical, mental, spiritual, emotional, and social), treat patients as their equals, give patients freedom to make choices, encourage patients to share in making decisions and taking responsibility for their care, try to see the patient's perspective, and place the patient's illness in a positive light.

Creating a Healing Sense of Place

Since the 1970s, there has been a strong revival of humanistic studies in the social sciences. In geography, this has led to an emphasis on sense of place, which has to do with the meanings that places have for people or that they give to places (Ley 1981). Meaning is achieved through the experiences people have in places. The kinds of meanings that places give people include a sense of identity, of security, of belonging (Pred 1983); places are where people find employment and social support, where they find aesthetic pleasure and feelings of pride. A sense of place can be established within one's house or a room in a house, within institutions such as schools and churches, even at work. As a healing example, one of the reasons for mental illness is a feeling of *rootlessness*, of no place to call home. Therefore, psychiatric patients benefit from *rootedness* or attachment to certain places (Godkin 1980).

The humanist geographer Yi-Fu Tuan gives us another perspective on sense of place when he talks about two contrasting elements that enhance our experience of place—public symbols and fields of care (Tuan 1974). *Public symbols*, Tuan says, appeal to the visual sense and are, perhaps, what strike us first about a place. Public symbols such as imposing hospital structures are often important in enhancing the reputation of a health care facility. Like St. Paul's Cathedral in London or the Empire State Building in New York, these public monuments make people feel proud of a place. Public symbols, however, can also be negative, such as when a building does not fit in with the surrounding architecture or is stigmatized by the community (e.g., a mental hospital).

Fields of care provide a more subtle and also, perhaps, a longer lasting attachment to place. This element, Tuan says, is appreciated by the non-visual senses and involves networks of interpersonal concern. It does not make an immediate impact, as public symbols do; rather, it is only felt after long experience. Of course we consider healing places to be fields of care; we look for them all our lives (Meyer and Cromley 1989). We remember the sound of the ocean at a beach retreat, the therapeutic touch of a nurse, or the kindly voice of a caring physician.

There are many reasons why people become attracted to a place because they believe it will heal them physically, mentally, spiritually, emotionally, and socially. It may be the natural beauty or tranquility that one remembers about a favorite spot; or the buildings that provide a sense of solidity and security; or the symbolic meaning of such things as the statue of a local hero; or remembering the support one had in a particular place from family and friends. This list is based on the kinds of things that I found to be important in the three healing places discussed in this book; each item represents an aspect of an "environment" that contributed to a healing sense of place.

Healing Environments

The main argument of this book is that places achieve a healing sense of place because several different, but often related, types of environments have been created there. This argument arises out of a body of work, mainly carried out by health geographers over the past ten years, that deals with the topic of "therapeutic landscapes." An article published in 1992 set out some ideas about factors that might be involved in creating therapeutic landscapes (Gesler 1992). The concept was used by others as a way to theorize or provide a framework for their work. In 1998 Robin Kearns and I edited a book titled *Putting Health into Place: Landscape, Identity, and Well-Being* that attempted to capture new ways of thinking and doing research in health geography. The first section contained papers on therapeutic landscapes in three places: Bath, England; Hot Springs, South Dakota; and Chile. The following year Allison Williams edited a book with the title *Therapeutic Landscapes: The Dynamic between Place and Wellness*, based partly on papers presented at a medical/health geography conference. The book was composed of chapters related to three themes: healing places; therapeutic environments and marginalized people; and symbolic landscapes in health care systems. In the past several years, several articles and book chapters have also picked up on the therapeutic landscape theme. The books and articles extended the idea in several new directions, well beyond the focus of this book, which is on specific places that achieved a lasting reputation for healing. The term "healing places" that forms the title of this book is a subset of a more comprehensive "therapeutic landscape" idea.

I found that therapeutic landscape ideas can best be operationalized by thinking in terms of several healing environments. I also believe that it is necessary to take a very wide, interdisciplinary, and eclectic view of the concept of environment when dealing with healing places. There are many reasons why people feel a strong attachment to place; these reasons and their relative importance vary from site to site and person to person. Perhaps the most commonly accepted notion of an environment is "nature" or one's natural surroundings, so we will certainly include the *natural environment*. Buildings and other human-made constructions are also a commonly accepted part of our surroundings; they constitute what we will call the *built environment*. The remaining two environments considered in this book are perhaps not as obvious as the natural and built ones, although I hope to demonstrate their significance as well. People are often strongly affected by either the concrete or abstract symbols they experience in places; this fact leads to the inclusion of the *symbolic environment* in our list. In any healing situation, the people involved (patients, doctors, nurses, technicians, managers) play various social roles and must interact with each other in a variety of ways. In other words, social relationships are important, the *social environment* affects a healing sense of place. There is obvious overlap between these environments; for example, important symbols may be derived from nature. However, for the sake of analysis, the environments are distinguished here.

I found all of these four environments—natural, built, symbolic, and social—to be important to the healing reputations of three places—Epidauros in Greece, Bath in England, and Lourdes in France—albeit in different ways (see below for how these three places were chosen for study). The final list of four environments, came about after working through the three case study locations and represents what is common to all of them. Table 1.1 lists several important aspects of the four environments.

Natural Environments

We know that many, if not most, societies around the world believe that nature has healing powers. For example, in eighteenth- and nine-teenth-century England, pastoral and romantic poetry extolled the restorative powers of nature (Gold 1985). Reacting to William Blake's "dark satanic mills" of the Industrial Revolution, poets such as William Wordsworth wrote of finding healing in the meadows, woods, and moun-tains of the countryside. In *Lines Composed a Few Miles above Tintern Abbey*, he wrote, "[I am] well pleased to recognize / In nature and the lan-guage of the sense, / The anchor of my purest thoughts, the nurse, / The guide, the guardian of my heart and soul / Of all my moral being" (Wordsworth 1975, 41).

Many people feel that they can attain physical, mental, and spiritual healing simply by spending time out-of-doors or seeking out remote or isolated places where they can "get away from it all," surrounded by undis-turbed nature. This idea is behind the *biophilia hypothesis*, which states that as humans evolved they acquired an affinity for nature and therefore feel comforted by it (Kellert and Wilson 1993). In the urbanized Western

Table 1.1   Aspects of Healing Environments

Environment	Aspects
Natural	Belief in nature as healer
	Beauty, aesthetic pleasure
	Remoteness, immersion in nature
	Specific elements of nature
Built	Sense of trust and security
	Affects the senses
	Pride in building history
	Symbolic power of design
Symbolic	Creation of meaning
	Physical objects as symbols
	Importance of rituals
Social	Equality in social relations
	Legitimization and marginalization
	Therapeutic community concept
	Social support

world an ideology has developed that extols the restorative powers of rural life in contrast to the pollution and stresses of the city (Marx 1968; Williams 1973). For example, the preferred locations for insane asylums in nineteenth-century England were in the countryside (Edginton 1997; Philo 1987). Nowadays, stressed-out company executives are sold "ecotherapy" weeks in natural settings.

In addition to a generalized feeling that nature heals, there are several specific elements taken from nature that are held to possess healing powers. Water is probably the most important of these elements; not only does it cleanse the body, it cleanses the soul (Parker 1983). It is hard to think of a place famous for healing that is not associated with a mineral spring, a stream, a river, or a lake; Vance (1972) and Cayleff (1988), who write of the search for healing waters in the United States, are just two of the many scholars who have studied these healing places. Other aspects of nature are also deemed to be important to health. In parts of Africa, Central America, and the American South, geophagy, or the ingestion of certain types of earth, is believed to meet both physiological and psychological needs (Hunter 1973; Hunter, Horst, and Thomas 1989). Some people think that bees have special healing powers (Lawrence 1993), and recent studies demonstrate the comfort animals bring to people who are ill (for example, see Beck 1986). Looking at or working in gardens is also considered to have a therapeutic effect; currently there are many experimental gardening programs in psychiatric hospitals and children's and senior's centers that are believed to have the potential to heal (Chadwick 1997; Gerlach-Spriggs, Kaufman, and Warner 1998) (see figure 1.1). A recent segment on National Public Radio described the planting of around a million daffodils in New York City parks as a "healing garden."

It is clear that there is a widespread belief that nature heals and of course that belief is important because it can affect one's health. But is there clinical proof that nature heals? There is, of course, abundant evidence that the parts of plants that make up the pharmacopoeia of both traditional and modern medical systems can effectively treat many ailments (Ayensu 1981; Plotkin 1993). But there is also empirical evidence that exposure to nature is therapeutic (Ulrich et al. 1991). For example, a well-known scientific experiment involved the ability of hospital patients to see (or not see) a stand of trees from their window (Ulrich 1984). Patients

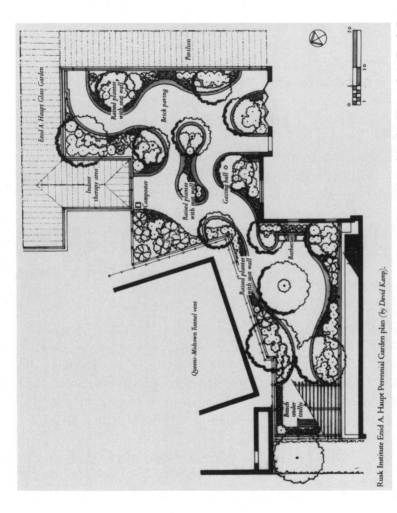

Rusk Institute Enid A. Haupt Perennial Garden plan (*by David Kamp*).

Figure 1.1. Rusk Institute Enid A. Haupt Perennial Garden Plan. This garden is found at the Howard A. Rusk Institute of Rehabilitative Medicine in lower Manhattan, New York City. Dr. Rusk built this restorative garden at his hospital as part of his goal to treat the whole person. From Nancy Gerlach-Spriggs, Richard Enoch Kaufman, and Sam Bass Warner Jr., *Restorative Gardens: The Healing Landscape* (New Haven, Conn.: Yale University Press, 1998), 58. This image appears courtesy of Yale University Press.

recovering from cholecystectomy (gall bladder surgery) who could see the trees had shorter postoperative stays, received fewer negative comments in nurses' notes, and took fewer patent analgesics compared to a matched group of patients who looked out on a brick wall.

Built Environments

The human-made or built environment has been shown to affect the healing process. Florence Nightingale (1863) recognized this when she discussed, among several other specific items, the importance to hospital patients of low ward densities, circulation of fresh air, adequate light, good drainage, clean laundry rooms and kitchens, and good accommodations for nursing staff. The hygienic standards that she introduced in her work in London, Scutari (during the Crimean War), and India during the nineteenth century saved thousands of lives.

Much of the scientific study of the effects of the built environment on health has been conducted by environmental psychologists (e.g., see Bagley 1974; Holahan 1979; Reizenstein 1982). Their guiding idea is that what people experience from their surroundings affects their moods and emotions and the ways in which they act. Spencer and Blades (1986) have argued for the importance of the supporting, controlling, and competitive roles played by building designs (buildings as a whole and rooms within buildings) on human behavior. Most aspects of human-made environments affect the senses; in fact, most hospital patients tend to rate the importance of what they can see, hear, smell, taste, and feel relatively highly (Hutton and Richardson 1995). Some studies have been carried out on the effects of different types of hospital designs. Verderber (1986) discussed patient perceptions of a continuum of hospital designs from those with windowless rooms to those with rooms having many windows. Kenny and Canter (1979) questioned nurses about their reactions to three hospital ward designs: radial, double corridor, and single corridor; their survey included items on efficiency and comfort both at specific locations within wards and in the ward as a whole.

The examples just given indicate that the effects on health of the built environment can often be studied quantitatively. However, health care facilities and other constructions may have less tangible effects that can only be looked at qualitatively. The imposing architecture of a hospital may create a feeling of confidence and trust; a recent example is the successful effort by a group of concerned citizens to save St. Bartholomew's Hospital in London. The architecture of York Retreat, a small private asylum in Yorkshire built by William Tuke in 1796, came to represent ideas about "moral treatment" and influenced the design of late nineteenth-century asylums (Edginton 1997). Even a mental hospital that has been stigmatized by a community can still have a nostalgic appeal for former patients following deinstitutionalization (Cornish 1997).

Symbolic Environments

The two environments discussed so far—natural and built—are relatively easy to grasp because they are tangible or accessible to the five senses. And yet, when we try to connect these environments to healing, we are forced to think of what they might *mean*. What meaning, for example, does having a water fountain on the grounds of a hospital have for a healing sense of place? Abstract ideas, such as beliefs about the best way to treat diabetes, also have meaning. These ideas about meaning lead one to consider a third healing environment, the symbolic one. Many of the objects we see around us or the ideas that people express have meaning because they symbolize something important in our lives. One cannot understand fully a person's reactions to an environment unless one recognizes that there are cognitive or symbolic mediators between stimulus and response (Evans 1982). The flag may evoke patriotic fervor, a crescent or cross may inspire religious veneration, and beliefs about what causes cancer may frighten us. Many anthropologists, as well as other social scientists, take the view that the physical and built environments we live in are products of symbolic actions (Daniels and Cosgrove 1988; Rowntree and Conkey 1980). Donald Meinig (1979, 6) writes, "We regard all landscapes as symbolic, as expressions of cultural values, social behavior, and individual actions worked upon particular localities over a span of time." These scholars tell us that we can learn to "read" environments for their symbolism, for what they tell us about people's thoughts and behaviors.

How do symbols work in healing? Arthur Kleinman suggests that they connect or mediate between biophysical and sociocultural worlds. In his words, "Healing occurs along a symbolic pathway of words, feelings, values, expectations, beliefs, and the like which connect events and forms with affective and physiological processes" (1973, 210). When someone is ill, the person tries to explain how he or she feels by using culturally encoded signs. Those who treat the person—family, friends, medical practitioners—attempt to read these signs, using either similar or different symbol systems.

There are other more specific examples of the foregoing ideas. The way mentally ill people are thought of or treated is in a large degree dependent on symbolic representations of them that are culturally based (e.g., they are "deviants," "a threat to society," or "children" to be taken care of) (Clark and Dear 1984). The Qollahuaya Indians, who live in the Bolivian Andes, have developed a complex system of symbolic pathways between the topography and hydrologic cycles of the mountains in which they live and their own bodies. They believe that, just as the health of a mountain depends on the circulation of water, human health depends on the proper distribution of air, blood, fat, and other materials throughout the body (Bastien 1985).

The easiest symbols to look for are physical objects. Earlier, we talked about what water symbolizes in healing places: divine blessing, purity, absolution, washing out sin and disease. The physician's white coat may be associated with purity or honesty (Blumhagen 1979). For many people, the high-tech equipment they see in modern hospitals symbolizes the power of biomedicine; although they may fear some machines, they put their trust in them (Kenny and Canter 1979).

Abstract symbols also provide meaning to healing situations. Rituals often contain symbolic language or actions that celebrate, maintain, and renew one's world as well as deal with its dangers (Helman 1994). On a simple level, a doctor may aid healing by using a simple, ritual phrase such as "You're going to be all right; it just takes time," which the patient wants and expects to hear. Many healing ceremonies (e.g., among Native Americans) contain ritual language that is intended to transform the patient from sickness to health (Tambiah 1968). Among the Qollahuaya mentioned above, social health depends on rituals that mix products produced by three levels of communities (corresponding to location at different heights on the mountainside) in a central place and then redistribute them up and down the mountain (Bastien 1985). Csordas (1983), examining the healing rituals of Catholic Pentecostals in the United States, showed that patients were transformed by meaningful and convincing discourses. Although the ritual did not always remove symptoms, it changed the meanings patients attached to illness or changed people's lifestyles.

Myths, which are symbolic stories, have been used in many societies to explain the world and provide models for behavior. Religious healers, shamans, and psychotherapists can use myths to heal; as an example, a shaman used a story about heroes who undertook a perilous journey, stopping at places analogous to sites along the birth canal, to help a woman come through a difficult childbirth (Dow 1986). A myth has been used to treat diabetes and alcoholism, which have a high prevalence among the Ojibway of southern Ontario. The story draws its lesson from a contrast between Nanabush, the teacher who represents truth in Ojibway legend, and the gluttonous Windigo, who symbolizes inappropriate responses to environmental stress as well as the symptoms of diabetes. The myth has healing power because it resonates with Ojibway beliefs that spiritual strength is necessary to health, and that there are correspondences between imbalances within the body, within society, and between people and the physical environment (Hagey 1984).

The stories that people tell about their illnesses and those of others may have strong symbolic force. Listening carefully to these illness narratives may reveal what people really believe about such things as what caused their problem or what should be done about it (Kleinman 1988). As an example, native healers among both the Cuna Indians of Panama and the Malays of Malaysia use birth narratives, which employ metaphors used in everyday speech, to help women through difficult childbirth (Laderman 1987). Price's experience from listening to misfortune tales told about illness by people in a marginal, mostly mestizo neighborhood of Quito, Ecuador, led her to state that illness stories "encode cultural models of causation, extensive situation knowledge about appropriate behavior when someone is sick, and a vast amount of cultural knowledge about types of treatment and health specialists" (1987, 313).

Social Environments

Healing is a social activity, it involves interactions among people who are playing various social roles. For example, many actors come together in the building of a hospital. I own a print by H. Stodard, copied from an original painting by the nineteenth-century artist Matthew Ward. It depicts The Royal Hospital Chelsea for veterans of the regular army who were no longer able to serve either because of poor health or length of service. The print does not focus on the hospital building itself. Rather, it represents the social context in which it was built and the actors deemed to be most important. Pictured are Charles II, king and patron who founded the hospital in 1682; an unidentified lady; Sir Christopher Wren, the most famous architect of his day; and a humble pensioner. The quality of social relationships in health care settings is important. What is particularly important for healing is that there be equality between healer and healed, feelings of mutual respect and trust. Unfortunately, relationships between individuals or groups of people are often characterized by dominance on one side and submission on the other (Eyles and Woods 1983); this is certainly the case in the field of medicine. Many people, in fact, see biomedicine as a major institution that is used to control people's lives (Zola 1972). Physicians and other medical people exercise a great deal of power over our lives through their authority to diagnose ills and prescribe treatments. There is also a dominance hierarchy within medical practice itself, with specialist physicians, primary care physicians, physician's assistants, nurses of different grades, lab technicians, and others all assigned their places.

However, attempts to dominate and control are often met with resistance (Jackson 1989). Scholars such as Illich (1976) and Navarro (1974) have criticized the hegemony imposed on medical practice by biomedicine in many places. In the nineteenth century, the hydrotherapy movement, which was in part a reaction to the dominance of physicians in health care delivery, helped women take control of their bodies (Cayleff 1988). Attempts were made to demystify such events as menstruation and childbearing by approaching them as natural processes as opposed to illnesses. Currently, the revival of alternative medical practices in the United States is, in some respects, a struggle against the dominance of the medical model (Gordon, Nienstedt, and Gesler 1998). Discontented with the inability of biomedicine to treat many illnesses, especially chronic diseases, and angered at uncaring attitudes, millions of Americans are spending large sums of money on chiropractors, homeopaths, New Age remedies, herbal teas, and a wide range of other nonbiomedical treatments.

Along with attempts to dominate come attempts to *legitimize* oneself and *marginalize* others. As a case in point, biomedicine struggled throughout the late nineteenth-century and well into the twentieth to support its own claims to medical authority and push alternatives such as chiropractors and homeopaths to the fringe (Gevitz 1988). The Flexner Report of 1910 had the effect desired by many physicians of cutting down competition from alternative healers. Another example is provided by Janzen (1978), who shows how native doctors, healing prophets, and practitioners of biomedicine in the Congo struggled throughout the twentieth century to legitimize themselves and marginalize their rivals.

Another aspect of control, in medicine as in other spheres of life, is the development of *ideologies* that promote the interests of a dominant group (Jackson 1989; Krause 1977). Ideologies often become "common sense" and may mask the true intentions of a controlling group. One specific example is the definition of alcoholism and drug addiction as illnesses as opposed to personal moral dilemmas (Staiano 1979). Another example is the promotion of the desirability, if not the absolute necessity, of using expensive high-tech equipment in hospitals or telemedicine services in rural areas, as part of an ideology that resonates with the importance of the "machine" metaphor that is very prevalent in modern society (Mills 1982).

The idea that good social relationships are essential to providing healing environments was at the core of the *therapeutic community* or *milieu therapy* movement that began in World War II (Filstead and Rossi 1973); attempts were made to break down hierarchies and divisions between patients and staff and develop full participation within a community atmosphere (Manning 1989). Moos (1977b) used the notion of a *social climate* to express these kinds of ideas and attempted to measure the phenomenon in hospital settings. The concepts of a therapeutic community and a social climate will be taken up again in chapter 5 on hospitals.

Choosing Healing Places to Study

The choice of places to research came at the end of a process that began with thinking about what constitutes healing and a healing sense of place, and which healing environments contribute to healing places. These ideas and the logic of their connections seemed plausible, but how valid were they? The next stage was to look for places that had achieved a lasting reputation for healing and examine them in the light of healing environments.

One faces a problem when looking for specific healing places to study and write about. Healing environments can be found almost anywhere; each person has places they would or would not like to be when they are sick and trying to recover. I wanted to know if there were places that many people found to have healing power over a fairly long period of time. Of course there were. Everyone has their favorite, so choices had to be made. Asked about healing places in casual conversation, several people mentioned spas, whether in Europe, North America, Japan, or other places around the world. This led to the choice of Bath, once known as the premier English watering place, as a good choice for a place to both visit and write about. As well as claiming curative powers for its mineral springs, this town was famous for its Georgian architecture, a myth about a healing king, and a colorful and complex social life. Then a colleague who found out about my interest in therapeutic landscapes suggested Epidauros in Greece where, for a thousand years, the human/god Asclepius healed people in dreams, so I researched and visited this healing place as well. Epidauros's attractions included a remote location amid gently rolling hills, masterpieces of sacred Greek architecture, legends about Asclepius, and a reputation for treating patients with different backgrounds equally. Finally, looking for a place that was established relatively recently and was still an active healing site, I hit upon Lourdes in France. After reading about this Marian pilgrimage place, I joined a pilgrim group and spent five days there. Among other things, Lourdes has a beautiful natural setting at the foot of the Pyrenees, a dynamic tension between built sacred and profane spaces, a pervading religious faith in healing, and a strong sense of community belonging.

The three chapters that follow this introductory chapter are based, in large part, on a reworking of earlier studies of the three places (Gesler 1993, 1996, 1998). These pieces were written over a span of about six years and represent an evolution of thinking about healing places. For the purposes of this book, Epidauros, Bath, and Lourdes are described as having a healing sense of place in terms of the four environments outlined above in order to present a coherent set of narratives. I will show that the theoretical points made in this chapter have solid empirical referents. Although all three places are similar because they fall within the traditions of Western culture, they achieved their reputations for healing in very diverse times and places. So we can expect that the details of how they exemplify environmental themes will be different. At the same time, I hope to show that the underlying ideas are really the same in all three places. Furthermore, one should always keep in mind that the four environments are contributing toward a very strong healing sense of place. Finally, the descriptions should lead the reader to think about applications of the ideas to modern health care institutions, the subject of chapter 5 on hospitals. The hospital chapter is intended to show that healing environments can both be found and created today. In fact, there is a surprising amount of literature on hospital design and creating therapeutic environments in hospitals that can be organized into the four healing environments discussed in detail above. This, I believe, is an encouraging sign.

Conclusion

The main argument of this chapter, and indeed the entire book, is that place matters to health. This of course is a major tenet of health geography, but it has also been acknowledged by a wide variety of people interested in the delivery of health care, whether explicitly or not. Today's reemerging interest in hospital design certainly recognizes that the environments of a place that has the potential to heal are important.

There is a tendency to think that current health problems can only be solved by employing current thinking. This attitude fails to recognize the influence of the past on what people's thinking is now. The bulk of this book provides evidence about four healing environments in three places that achieved lasting reputations for healing. Because the geographic and historical context of each of these places is unique, I do not advocate applying specific features of these environments to modern health care situations. Rather, it is the general ideas that I strongly believe can be adapted to current situations. In a sense, the book provides an organizing framework for many ideas that are currently being put into practice.

Of course there are limitations to a study of this type. First, there are only three case studies, certainly not enough for any statistical analysis of "healing factors." But to me the admittedly largely anecdotal evidence is compelling, especially as the same kinds of environments were found to be important in all three places. Second (and colleagues have pointed this out more than once), the examples are based on Western sites. There is much to be learned from non-Western places, too. An excellent example is the Navajo, whose entire homeland is a therapeutic landscape in their eyes (Dobbs 1997). I would still argue that non-Western healing places may usefully be examined in the light of the four environments, however. Third, the idea of healing places can be extended beyond the specific sites dedicated to healing discussed in this book to places associated with the maintenance of health and well-being. These places could include, as examples, the home of an elderly person receiving home health care or an office building.

A fourth limitation of the book is that it says little about the contested nature of healing places. Put most simply, what is a healing environment for one individual or group may not be for another. The hospital design process, for example, is a contentious one. Reading about healing places may give one the impression that all that has to be done is to think positively about certain features of healing landscapes and put them into place. But this approach avoids many important questions (Bell 2001). Where does the knowledge that is brought to creating healing environments come from? In the case of this book, it comes from my reading of various accounts about three historical Western places, but others could disagree with my findings. Who has the power to say what healing environment features will be put into practice? Who is allowed to participate in creating therapeutic environments? And how do the various groups of people who are supposed to benefit from healing places interpret various features, experience them, feel about them? In other words, how do the various "cultures" (defined by gender, ethnicity, position in the hospital hierarchy, and so on) react to specific healing environments? Although these questions are touched upon to some extent in the book, they are not dealt with explicitly as they are beyond the scope of the present task, which is to present "successful" examples of healing places.

~~

CHAPTER TWO

Epidauros: Asclepius and Dream Healing

For a thousand years people came to a remote spot in ancient Greece, the sanctuary of Epidauros, believing that the god Asclepius, son of Apollo and a human mother, Koronis, would appear to them in dreams and heal them. Over time, this place became one of the most important centers in a vast network of Asclepian healing sites. How did Epidauros achieve and maintain a reputation that lasted from the fourth century B.C. to the sixth century A.D.? What contributed to its very strong healing sense of place? My answer is, no single factor created and sustained this healing site. By telling the story of Epidauros in terms of the four environments developed in chapter 1—natural, built, symbolic, and social—I hope to show how several factors, working together, established its fame.

A Pleasing Solitariness

One attraction of Epidauros must have been its remoteness; patients seeking divine cures at the Epidaurian sanctuary in Greek or Roman times had to make a substantial effort to get there. Its setting was distinctly rural, a place where people could come directly into contact with untouched nature. Most visitors would have first traveled, by land or by sea, to the port town of Epidauros. This little place was located on the northern side of the Argive Peninsula, about thirty miles southwest of Athens across the Saronic Gulf, and about eighteen miles southeast of Corinth on the mainland of the Peloponnese (Tomlinson 1983) (figure 2.1). It wasn't far from these centers of Grecian power, but Epidauros, chief town of the Epidaurian state, was by no means an important place (Burford 1969). Indeed, the main attraction lay several miles away.

Within the relatively isolated Epidaurian state lay the isolated Asclepian sanctuary. It was a nine-mile trek by foot or on animal back, up into the hills to the southwest of the port. It took James G. Frazer, an anthropologist who made many other excursions into ancient rites and mysteries, two and one half hours to complete the ride in 1890. He found the scenery along his path to be rugged, but extremely beautiful. Using the hyperbole familiar to readers of nineteenth-century European travel literature, he wrote that he had passed through a "wild, romantic ravine," with the "lofty precipitous banks" of a stream towering on either side (Frazer 1898, 260). Coming upon the sanctuary in an open valley encircled by hills, he went on to say, "the whole scene has a certain pleasing solitariness about it." Thus the traveler, having left the crowded, dusty town behind, moved ever upward through a harsh, wild, and unbounded wilderness and then arrived at a bounded sanctuary, a refuge nestled within a softer landscape (figure 2.2). "Perhaps," as Allison Burford writes, "visions were only seen, and inspirations to found sanctuaries only imparted, in surroundings capable of inspiring wonder and giving shelter" (1969, 43).

Asclepieia, places where Asclepius was believed to heal, could be found throughout the ancient world, but exactly what kinds of physical or natural landscapes were they sited within? It would be possible to construct a map of possible sites, using what the Greeks themselves said about where temples of healing should be found or indeed were found. The author of *Airs, Waters, and Places,* a central volume among the Hippocratic writings, said that a pleasant climate, good water quality, and beautiful scenery were all conducive to good health (Burford 1969). Vitruvius (fl. first century B.C.) said that Asclepian sites should be healthy, near fresh springs of water, and away from pestilence. Plutarch (46–120 A.D.) says simply that Asclepian temples were to be found on clear, elevated places in rural areas (Edelstein and Edelstein 1945). In other words, the Greeks were thinking a lot like the planners

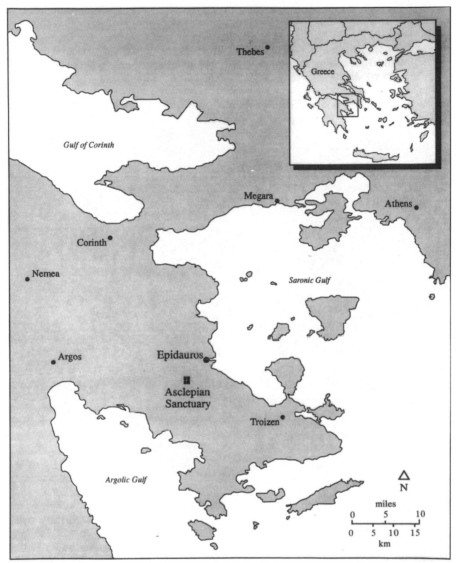

Figure 2.1.   Location of Epidauros and the Asclepian Sanctuary. The sanctuary lies in a secluded spot in rolling hills about eight miles from the coast of Greece and eighty miles from Athens, the Greek capital, by road. From W. M. Gesler 1993, "Therapeutic Landscapes: Theory and a Case Study of Epidauros, Greece," *Environment and Planning D: Society and Space* 11: 179 (London: Pion Limited). Reproduced with permission from Pion Limited.

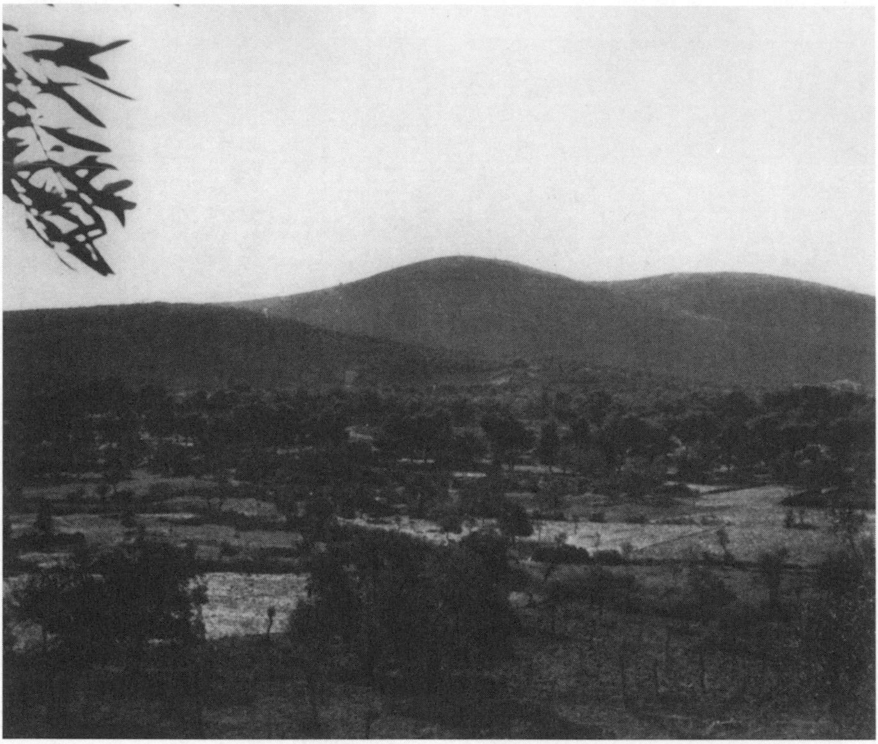

Figure 2.2.   A Pleasing Solitariness. The Asclepian sanctuary as seen from the north-west, looking toward the main temple area and the theater beyond. Note the gentle hills in the distance and the apparent stillness. From Alison Burford 1969, *The Greek Temple Builders of Epidauros* (Liverpool: University of Liverpool Press), p. 44. Reproduced with permission from Liverpool University Press.

of European and American insane asylums in the nineteenth century who followed a romantic notion of the healing powers of nature experienced in rural settings (Philo 1987). The siting of Epidauros certainly conformed to this ideal and probably contributed to the preeminence of the place. However, as is often the case, for many Asclepieia the Greek ideal and the real were quite different. Some were found on mountain tops, others in valleys, but more were sited within cities and towns than without (Stam and Spanos 1982). One was even founded in a swamp, despite the fact that some people were aware that the "miasmas" arising from such places were decidedly unhealthy. However, Epidauros itself maintained the ideal and this, I believe, helped it to maintain a dominant position among all the Asclepieia.

The site at Epidauros also gained a gift from nature that was vital to a land seldom blessed with rain: water. Water from springs was present at almost all Asclepian sanctuaries and we are told by the traveler Pausanius (who passed this way in the second century A.D.) that people were drawing water from a cistern at Epidauros when he visited there (Pausanius 1971). It was of course essential for the patients and staff to have a steady supply of water. Perhaps the water was drunk for medicinal purposes: water from two springs was analyzed early this century and found to have the same content as spring water in Evian, France. Water symbolizes many things connected with healing. Pouring forth from within the depths of the earth, it represents life and regeneration. And, with obvious relevance for the manner in which Asclepius healed, its flow is analogous to the cathartic action of dreams.

Water was an essential part of ritual purification at the sanctuary, just as it has been at sacred springs in many other places around the world. Pausanius says that there was a sacred fountain that was used for this purpose; a well and several shallow basins have also been unearthed at the site. Ritual purification was not merely a cleansing of the hands or other parts of the body (Parker 1983). To the Greeks it also symbolized a purification of the soul in preparation for communion with a god. There was a stone inscription at Epidauros that read: "He who enters the fragrant temple must be pure; purity is to think holy thoughts."

Purification was seen in opposition to pollution, which was associated with ritual impurity, unfitness to enter a temple, contagion, and danger that was not of secular origin (Parker 1983). The idea that disease could be washed away or purged out of the system was deeply embedded in the Greek psyche. So the drama of purification had a symbolic or psychological affect that dream healing, prayers, or diet could not rival. The Greeks, it should be noted, were not alone in having these kinds of beliefs. For example, Simon Schama claims that the proverbial cleanliness of the seventeenth-century Dutch went far beyond a concern for warding off decay and contagion (Schama 1988). He links Dutch ideas about cleanliness and filth to the polarities of pride and shame, solidarity and alienness, and claims that the Dutch burghers preached cleanliness to foster moral and social order among their subjects. The brooms and brushes that you can pick out in the paintings of the masters of that time, Schama says, represent Calvinist purity, sweeping history clean.

In reality, purification played a relatively little part in healing in the Asclepian temples, but there is evidence that many Apollonian and Asclepian cults grew up at the sites of sacred springs. In the Hippocratic writings there is the notion that the body is a container whose purification is naturally maintained by spontaneous purging such as excretion and menstruation. If a humor or vital principle was in excess within the body, disease occurred, and an artificial purification was required. Treatment might include "wiping off," fumigation, localized drenching, hot baths, or purgative drugs (Parker 1983). This sort of treatment is reminiscent of the "heroic medicine" still being practiced in the Western world in the nineteenth century. The interesting thing is that these secular methods of catharsis had religious connotations and so, despite the protestations of some Greek physicians that their medicine was different in kind from temple practice, the similarities could not be ignored. Certainly most lay people would hardly have quibbled over any perceived differences.

Asclepius's authority was greatly enhanced by his association with certain objects or elements in nature (Caton 1900; Frazer 1898; Kerenyi 1960; Meier 1967; Struckmann 1979). Animals are often featured in myths and symbolize powerful forces. Within the temple at Epidauros there was a statue of Asclepius, sitting on a throne, with a golden serpent rising up on his left hand, and a dog on his right. Frazer says that it is "tolerably certain" (1898, 65) that Asclepius was originally a serpent and was later turned into an anthropomorphic god with the serpent as his primary symbol. Snakes have been worshiped in many cultures and magical powers, including healing, have been attributed to them. Facts and beliefs about snakes reveal the reasons why they were thought to be so potent: they are said to be sharp-sighted and vigilant; a snake sheds its skin periodically, which symbolizes renewal of life, immortality, youth, the preservation of beauty, and the body's regeneration after illness; poisonous snakes have the power over life and death. To many of us, serpents are creatures to be feared and of course there is the association for the Christian world with evil deriving from the Garden of Eden story. The Greeks and Romans, however, were far more familiar with snakes than we are—they took them into their houses as domestic pets and, rather than keeping cats to get rid of mice, they used snakes. Noble Roman ladies, it is said, wrapped snakes around their necks to keep themselves cool. Perfectly harmless, fairly large (over four feet long) yellow snakes were common in the area around Epidauros; Pausanius (1971) says this species was only found here. The caduceus, which features two snakes curled around a staff with two wings at the top, remains a symbol of medical practice today.

One of the Asclepian myths says that after his birth he was guarded by a shepherd's dog. Dogs became associated with Asclepius and some were kept within the sanctuary. The ability of a dog to follow a trail and its intuitive powers were thought to be good qualities in a physician. Snakes and dogs, cure inscriptions (found carved on stones at the site) tell us, were involved in temple cures; for example, they licked people's wounds and sores. The cock, symbol of sunrise and radiance, was the most common animal to be slaughtered in homage to the god. Socrates, whose last words were, "Crito, we owe a cock to Asclepius; pay it and do not neglect it" (Edelstein and Edelstein 1945), was merely repeating a common phrase—interesting that he should say it as he passed from life over into the underworld.

An Ecology of Sacred Buildings

By the fourth century B.C. Asclepius's fame was on the rise and the number of visitors to the central shrine at Epidauros continued to rise as well. The leaders of the Epidaurian state stepped in to control the sanctuary, administered its affairs, and supervised a building program (Burford 1969; Tomlinson 1983). The head priest retained the title of chief official and controlled the treasury for some time, but later on the Epidaurian state appointed a board to handle the sanctuary's finances. The building commissioners and architects were probably appointed by the state, and two state bodies—the council and the assembly—decided what to build and how much to spend. An ambitious building program was launched and lasted for over a century. Stone and building materials were procured either locally or from outside the area, and a group of craftsmen and unskilled workers were recruited from all social classes.

With the exception of its well-preserved theater—which the guide books describe as one of the best examples, as well as one of the best preserved—in the ancient world, the buildings that were constructed at Epidauros have been leveled to the ground, either by the hand of nature or humans. However, we know a great deal about what the built environment of the site was like from two important sources. Fortunately, details about building design and building materials were carved in stone. Excavators have come across a set of large stones with inscriptions containing details such as the fact that a particular type of wood was purchased from a certain place at a certain time and for a specific price. These stones also contain the cure inscriptions mentioned above. In addition, we have the evidence of Pausanius, a traveler and writer who crisscrossed Greece in the second century A.D., and retold in his writings the multitude of stories he heard along the way (Habicht 1985).

Pausanius thought of himself as a historian, but he lacked the proper investigation into details concerning his sources—that is, he reported very interesting things, but they became encrusted with some obviously local biases. What he really seems to have had was the soul of a regional cultural geographer: he carved up Greece into districts and systematically journeyed from one to another, recording faithfully what he saw, what was written about places, and what people told him. What he lacked in historical accuracy he made up for in geographic exactitude. Heinrich Schliemann, the forceful nineteenth-century archaeologist, discoverer of ancient Troy, may be faulted for making surgical slices through multiple strata of ancient civilizations, eviscerating invaluable artifacts along the way, but where he had read Pausanius, he did his cutting in the right places. The excavations at Epidauros are one of many testimonies to Pausanius's accuracy and thoroughness (Habicht 1985).

If we take the evidence from stone inscriptions and Pausanius's accounts and then add in what is known about Greek architecture in general, we have a good idea of what many of the buildings at Epidauros looked like (figure 2.3). The first building a traveler, approaching the sanctuary along the ancient road up from Epidauros town, would have encountered was the Propylon, a formal, decorative entrance or gateway situated along the northern boundary. Since the boundary, a ring of stones, signified sacred ground within, the pilgrim who passed through the Propylon was making the transition from profane to sacred space (Tomlinson 1983). Within the sanctuary, some two dozen buildings, both

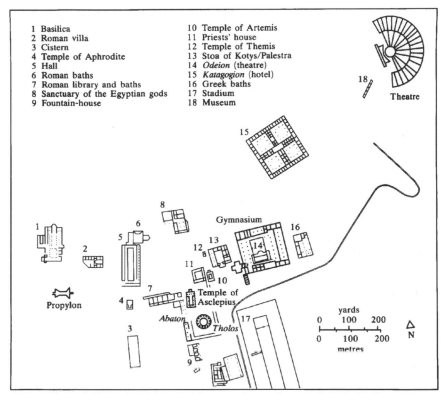

Figure 2.3.   A Plan of Epidauros. The map shows the complex of Greek and Roman buildings now seen at the site. The theater is one of the best preserved in the classical world. Healing focused on the Temple of Asclepius, the tholos, and the abaton. From W. M. Gesler 1993, "Therapeutic Landscapes: Theory and a Case Study of Epidauros, Greece," *Environment and Planning D: Society and Space* 11: 180 (London: Pion Limited). Reproduced with permission from Pion Limited.

Greek and Roman, were erected over several centuries. At the core was a trinity of buildings, the temple of Asclepius, the tholos, and the abaton, each with its distinctive architecture and, presumably, its unique function (although just what the tholos was for is still a matter of debate among scholars) (Burford 1969).

The temple was of conventional design and modest size, of the Doric order, with six columns in front and eleven along each side. The most beautiful building in the complex was the tholos, a circular building (a previously little-used shape in Greek architecture) that distinguished itself by having an outer Doric colonnade, an inner Corinthian colonnade, and a very finely decorated doorway. The abaton, a portico with an Ionic colonnade (completing the trinity of Grecian styles) about thirty-six meters long, was where the sick came to sleep and be healed by their god.

Vincent Scully writes, "the formal elements in any Greek sanctuary are, first, the specifically sacred landscape in which it is set and, second, the buildings that are placed within it" (1969, 1–2). This idea could be called "an ecology of sacred buildings" or, alternatively, "sermons in stones" because it indicates how human aspirations embodied in architecture interact with nature (which, for the Greeks, the gods produced) to raise a paean or song of praise to Asclepius. Each place where a temple complex was found had its own ecology, its unique configuration or grouping of buildings and topography. In the case of Epidauros, we have already spoken about the softness of the landscape that corresponded to Asclepius's gentle nature. The sanctuary's position in a hollow rather than on a mountaintop seems appropriate to a god lower in status than the principal Olympians. In a functional sense, the buildings embody the god because they were designed to house all the activities required for healing that had existed on the spot for centuries before. The buildings are, with the possible exceptions of the theater and the tholos, of modest proportion and simple style, which would accord with Asclepius's human scale and modesty. Perhaps we can go so far as to say that the dual human-god nature of Asclepius is represented in the temple and the tholos: the former, with its cult statue honors him as divine, and the latter, just as prominent within the core grouping, reflects him as mortal (Tomlinson 1983).

Much like a modern recreation center, there was a great deal for patients awaiting a summons to the abaton to do (and some waited up to four months until their auguries were favorable) (Caton 1900; Edelstein and Edelstein 1945; Tomlinson 1983). They could alternate between periods of rest and exercise. They could simply breathe in the fresh mountain air and take pleasure in wandering through the groves of trees outside the sanctuary. There was a library, a gymnasium, and a large theater for their use and entertainment. The well-preserved theater, in which the ancient comedies and tragedies are still acted out, is the ruin that attracts most tourists today. There must have been a thriving marketplace that catered to the demand for animal and other sacrifices—lucky the merchant who had a stall here and a guaranteed steady clientele.

Sacred Space, Dreams, and Healing Myths

Both concrete and abstract symbols may become an important part of a healing environment. How did symbolism play a role for visitors to Epidauros? For a start, the sanctuary was sited on sacred ground. Hallowed ground often has a long history; sacred places persist. We know that a sanctuary dedicated to Asclepius existed by the sixth century B.C., but religious practices carried out close to the site can be traced back to the Mycenaean Age, at its height around 1400 B.C. (Burford 1969). This was the Heroic Age, the Age of Homer, the age that spawned the myths about Olympian gods and epic wars. Sometime in the intervening centuries, a sanctuary on the slopes of a mountain was dedicated to Apollo, god of the sun. Asclepius, son of Apollo, settled in a spot somewhat lower, in a valley. What he and his followers lost in elevation, they gained back from a more accessible spot.

I would argue that the location of Epidauros was of symbolic importance. Earlier, I mentioned that most Asclepieia were located among concentrations of populations. These locations, it seems to me, rather than detracting from Asclepius's prestige, speak for his success. He began lower on the mountain than his father Apollo, spawned some rural temple complexes, and then moved down out of the hills altogether and into the daily lives of the congregations of people in the cities. He became more accessible by spreading out from the margins of political and social influence and into the cores. Meanwhile, at Epidauros, he maintained a position of preeminence, halfway between the mountain peaks above and the plains below.

The method of healing that Asclepius was said to have used in his Asclepieia was dream healing. For many societies, including modern industrial ones, dreams carry great symbolic force. Thus it is necessary to discuss healing dreams as an essential part of the symbolic environment at Epidauros. The ancient Greeks used four forms of divination, which are attempts to foretell the future or uncover hidden knowledge—interpretation of natural portents, the flight of birds, the entrails of sacrificial animals, and dreams (Hamilton 1906). Dream interpretation had the greatest vogue, so its application in Asclepian sanctuaries was nothing out of the ordinary. Therefore, most patients would have laid down in the abaton fully expecting to hear the god's voice, see mystical lights, or witness an apparition or epiphany of Asclepius. We know that many societies in ancient times shared this interest in dreams. Perhaps the most well-known example is Joseph's economic interpretation of the Egyptian Pharaoh's dream recorded in the Old Testament, with its practical meaning: the Egyptians must store up grain from fat times to prepare for lean days ahead. The Greeks believed that when people were asleep the soul was freed from the body so that it could soar into spiritual realms and commune with the gods. Dreams were divine revelations. People tried to induce dreams by entering into sacred places, performing the prescribed rituals, and then sleeping in a special place, a practice known as *incubation*. Seeking cures for disease was the most common reason for incubation, but any problem such as a financial worry or a family quarrel, could be brought for solution.

"Accurate knowledge about the signs which occur in dreams will be found very valuable for all purposes," says a Hippocratic writer and goes on to detail some of the commonly held beliefs about the nature of dreams and dream interpretation (Lloyd 1983, 252). In sleep, the soul performs all the functions of the body; it senses everything. If a person dreams of normal daytime thoughts and actions, that person is healthy, but if the dream runs contrary to the things that people normally do from day to day, this signals a disturbance. It is good to see the sun, moon, and stars, all in their right places, but if the heavenly bodies are out of place, wander, or are changed, then the dreamer has a disease. Disease in turn seems to have been a metaphor for deviation from or violation of the natural order of things in the body, in society, and in the cosmos.

To summarize the beliefs about dream healing that patients brought to Epidauros, one could say that they lived in a society where philosophers, physicians, and lay people all believed in the ability of dreams to help people in various ways. Medical knowledge about what causes illness and what cures were most effective was shared by patient, priest, and physician. Most people believed in divine intervention in healing and other spheres of life. Thus when people went to sleep in the abaton they shared common expectations about what might happen. They expected to see the god and they saw him; they expected to be told certain things and they were. Their dreams, in short, were based on everyday experiences, magnified by divine associations. The special atmosphere, the physical and mental environment, probably enhanced suggestibility, but what was suggested was already there. Secular medicine was prescribed, but was efficacious both because it had some intrinsic merit and people believed in it.

I believe that it is very important that when Asclepius flourished at Epidauros he was thought to be a god and yet he also retained human qualities; that is, he symbolized both the superhuman and human and thus provided a bridge between or mediated between two worlds. Paralleling the location of the sanctuary halfway between the mountains above and the plains below, Asclepius was half-human and half-divine. How could this be? A myth or symbolic story helps us to understand this seeming paradox. The most common version of Asclepius's story has been given the imprimatur of authority by a trio of the ancient world's greatest poets: Hesiod in his *Theogeny* around the eighth century B.C., Pindar (c. 522–440 B.C.) in his *IIIrd Pythian Ode* and Ovid (43 B.C.–17 A.D.) in *Metamorphoses*. The myth goes like this (Edelstein and Edelstein 1945; Papastamou 1977; Struckmann 1979; Tomlinson 1983). Apollo took as a lover Koronis, who was the daughter of King Phlegyas of Trikka in Thessaly. While the sun god was away at the sanctuary of Delphi, he instructed a white raven to keep an eye on his human consort. However, the raven could not prevent his charge from being unfaithful with a mortal lover. The raven flew with this news to Apollo and the god in his anger caused the raven's feathers to turn black, a curse the bird carries to this day. Apollo told his sister Artemis what had happened and she killed Koronis, pregnant now with Apollo's child. But, as Koronis was about to be consumed on her funeral pyre, her lover god, full of remorse, brought forth the child Asclepius alive from his mother's womb. Hesiod claimed that this event was the first recorded Cesarean birth in European history.

Apollo placed his son under the care of Cheiron, a wise centaur, who educated him to become a great physician. Cheiron himself was an interesting and ambiguous hybrid. His animal body represented the destructiveness of nature and yet he instructed humans in medicine and music. Although a god, he suffered from an incurable wound. Perhaps this contradiction, like those of Asclepius, represents the contradictions of medicine: the wounder and the wounded heal.

Asclepius was a great physician but, like so many Greek heroes and gods, he had a fatal flaw. He was greedy, and for the sake of money dared to heal those who were doomed to die. Once he went too far and restored the dead Hippolytos to life. Zeus, father of the gods, became angry at this and struck and killed Asclepius with a thunderbolt. Later, the extraordinary physician himself was brought back to life and became a god.

Now we have an easy solution to our puzzle about Asclepius's status: he has mixed parentage, a human mother and a divine father. Like Jesus Christ, he somehow connects the human and the divine. Is that all there is to it? I would suggest not. Stories of the gods and other extraordinary people and events exist on two levels: the level of manifest meaning, the *problem*, and the level of hidden or latent meaning, the *riddle* (Walter 1988). Take one of the most well known of the Greek tragic stories, the tale of "Oedipus the King," as illustration. Thebes was desolated by a pestilence, a disease that was personified by the monster Sphinx who brooded over the city. The city could be released from its bondage to sickness only if someone could answer a riddle that the wily Sphinx posed. "What creature," the Sphinx asked, "goes on four in the morning, on two at noon, and on three in the evening?" When Oedipus replied, "Man," the Sphinx threw itself to destruction and the city was saved. The answer of the future king is neat and clever; it solves the problem. But there is also a deeper meaning that relates each stage of life to the earth and sky: humans crawl on the ground as the sun rises; they walk upright when the sun is overhead; they lean back down toward the earth as the sun goes down. Thus they are connected with nature and with the universe. On the level of the riddle, the spirit of disease disappears when people remember their proper relationship with the universe. This is the message of the conservationist, told three millennia ago.

The manifest or problem meaning of the Asclepian myth lies in his mixed parentage. On this level, we also have a typical story of the unseemly behavior of the gods that, like a distorting mirror at a fair, makes large the passions of everyday life (Edelstein and Edelstein 1945). Under this interpretation, we witness crimes (unfaithfulness and murder), passion between lovers (Koronis and her two paramours) remorse (Apollo repents), greed (Asclepius desires wealth), a Promethean-like challenge to the gods and to the order of things (Asclepius dares to raise the dead), reaction by the gods (Zeus darts his fatal thunderbolt), and redemption/resurrection (Asclepius ascends to godhead). To look beyond this level of everyday drama writ large, we are guided by the idea that myths are a response to apparently intolerable or refractory experiences such as illness or death, which no one understands completely. Pausanius shows his understanding of this idea:

> When I began this work I used to look on these Greek stories as little better than foolishness; but now that I have got as far as Arcadia my opinion about them is this: I believe the Greeks who were accounted wise spoke of old in riddles and not straight out; and, accordingly, I conjecture that this story about Crossus is a bit of Greek philosophy. (Habicht 1985, quote from Pausanius, VIII, 8.3)

Just what is the bit of Greek philosophy in Asclepius's tale? For a start, we may take Asclepius's birth in his mother's death as a symbol of healing itself. I also suggest that the mortal/god represents both the opportunities and restraints associated with the practice of medicine. Asclepius has extraordinary powers to heal, and this is an inspiration to the medical profession and to humankind in general. On the other hand, if mortals overreach themselves in their hunger for money or attempt to usurp supernatural powers, they are doomed to fail and will inevitably be struck down.

Social Relations between Healers and Healed

We can gain a great deal of insight about healing at Epidauros if we examine the interactions between the Greek people, their doctors, Asclepius, and the temple priests at the sanctuary (Edelstein and Edelstein 1945; Lloyd 1979; Nutton 1985). In other words, the social environment or context of social relationships was important to the healing process. We begin with a look at patient/doctor relationships in Grecian times. Secular physicians were in a rather precarious position. Doctors themselves had little to say about who could or should be called a physician; the decision was mainly up to the public. The definition of "doctor" was usually simple and pragmatic; someone could claim the title if they carried out medical treatment for a fee or gifts and devoted most of their time to healing. The status of physicians was relatively low; in fact, they were considered to be on the same level as tradesmen. Even if an educated person became interested in medicine and became quite proficient in its practice, it was a rare thing to stoop to calling oneself a doctor. Indeed, this was the situation in the Western world not much longer than a century ago.

Medical information was relatively accessible among the general population and there was a great deal of lay involvement in medical debates and practice. Self-medication, ignoring any medical advice, was common. This meant that interactions between patients and doctors were far more open and more on a basis of equality than is true in Western society today. Not surprisingly, this system spawned a large number of quacks, and many of them were exposed in time, which did little for the profession. And physicians had to compete with many others who professed to cure—the alternative healers of the day—herb cutters, druggists, midwives, diviners, gymnastic trainers, exorcists, and priests. At times physicians were subject to vicious attacks. The elder Pliny (23–79 A.D.), probably reflecting a widespread undercurrent of antiphysician sentiment, declared that the Greek medicine being practiced in his day was nothing less than wholesale murder that went unpunished.

Greek physicians, as they did in North America and Europe in the nineteenth and twentieth centuries, did not take this sort of abuse without fighting back. They recognized their plight and constantly struggled to earn respect, a sense of professionalism, and legitimization (Frede 1987; Lloyd 1979; Nutton 1985). On the religious front, they sought the patronage of Asclepius, a popular god. On the secular front, some doctors were strongly motivated to turn medicine into a scientific subject and gain prestige from the general respect accorded to rational thought. The problem was, many medical theories were often flimsy and not the kind of ideas that could be verified with controlled experiments. In contrast, many physicians made their reputations from careful observations and sound clinical practice. Others took advantage of the spirit of the day that appreciated rhetoric and the persuasive use of language and spoke eloquently to large audiences. The most successful added patients to their lists and perhaps even won posts as public physicians. But at the same time as they were trying to achieve more status as a group, physicians vied for status among themselves. Those doctors who could claim and demonstrate a greater knowledge and expertise through their words and deeds tried to distance themselves from the lower orders and marginalize other physicians.

The common people had a special relationship to Asclepius. For a start, he was a local god, which enhanced his accessibility. Here we encounter a paradox: Asclepius became known everywhere and yet he remained a local god. How was he local? Wherever he was enshrined, he became the genius loci of the place, much as the Virgin Mary in later times was venerated and took on the name of the places where she was seen in visions (e.g., "Our Lady of Lourdes"; see chapter 4). In each locality, Asclepius, unlike the national gods, the Olympians, was worshiped by people in their own way. He was "at home" in his temples, demonstrating his earthly powers from day to day (Meier 1967). And, although there is disagreement about the point, it seems that Asclepius was local in another way—he was a *chthonic* god, which means that he had gone down into the earth and become invested with its powers (Burford 1969; Hamilton 1906). The requisite artifacts and connections with the earth are there to support this contention: altars in Asclepian temples where burnt sacrifices were made and blood was spilled out onto the ground; the use of things arising from the earth—plants, animals, and minerals—in temple healing; and, again, the association between death and the underworld. All these associations with nature serve to reinforce the concept of Asclepius as chthonian god, linked closely to the earth and life arising out of death.

Asclepius appears to have had a universal appeal. He is described as kind and gentle and yet was imposing, too—he inspired awe. In Greek, his name can be translated as "the one who gently takes pains with the sick." Artists sculpted him or drew him as a venerable old man with a heavy beard and thick, wavy hair. However, in some descriptions he is given a dark side that kills, in contrast to his healing powers (Meier 1967). Perhaps this duality reflects the slender balance between life and death, illness and health.

Asclepius was in tune with the times (or the times were in tune with him, if that is how you look at history). By the end of the fifth century, the Greeks were beginning to express a craving for personal relationships with their gods (Edelstein and Edelstein 1945; Papastamou 1977). For many, the old pantheon, the Olympians, were too remote. What they wanted was someone divine and yet human enough to be concerned with them as individuals. Asclepius fit these requirements; he was a personality for the age.

The working poor, known as the "dusty feet," had reason to venerate Asclepius because he accepted every genuinely ill person into his sanctuaries and only asked from each according to their means (Stam and

Spanos 1982; Struckmann 1979). His temples inspired charity and became centers for the distribution of money and food. He offered a safety
net to the middle and lower classes that had little access to trained physicians or other forms of care. Many households included Asclepius among
their collection of gods (Edelstein and Edelstein 1945; Papastamou 1977;
Struckmann 1979). In fact, he was a family man himself. Homer speaks
of his twin sons: Podaleirios, an expert on internal diseases, and
Machaon, an expert surgeon. One of his daughters, Panacea, has left an
unfortunate legacy in her name, but far more respected now is Hygieia,
patron goddess of public health. It has been said that, since Asclepius was
famed as a curer only, Hygieia made her appearance in order to extend his
powers to prevention as well. Whether this is true or not, daughter and
father have been engaged in a centuries-long intra-family feud between
medicine and public health that is no more resolved today than it was
twenty-five hundred years ago (Dubos 1959).

Physicians, too, often sought close ties with Asclepius. Many physicians took Asclepius as their patron god (Edelstein and Edelstein 1945).
Here was a figure they could identify with on a human level, someone
who understood and practiced the same kind of medicine. At the same
time, his skills were extraordinary, supernatural in fact, and thus he
served as a prototype, an ideal toward which they could strive. More
practically, Asclepius was a person around whom physicians could rally;
that was very important in an age in which their status was low and subject to the whims of their clients. In other words, the healing god offered
legitimization.

Social relationships between healer and healed at the Epidaurian sanctuary itself must also be considered. Evidence points to its role as a social
leveler. We can see this by asking who came to the sanctuary and who was
permitted to come in. The sick gained entry of course, but also those who
were not and came to worship the god, those who wanted to stay well,
and those who simply wanted to join the daily round of activities. It was
said that Asclepius excluded no one, but, like any sacred place, there was
the real possibility that certain categories of people might be turned aside.
The uninitiated and the infidel are not always welcome at the holy
shrine. Indeed, at Epidauros, no one near death or close to giving birth
was allowed to cross through the gate that linked profane and sacred
ground (Caton 1900). One could be cynical and say that the temple

priests were conveniently eliminating the terminally ill and potentially difficult pregnancies. On the other hand, it also makes symbolic sense to exclude vital events that represent the endpoints of life from a place where preserving life was the ultimate goal.

It is easy to focus only on the dream healing that took place in the sanctuary at Epidauros (perhaps because they stimulate modern minds primed for psychoanalytic possibilities), but a great deal of bustle and noise went on during the day, which led to the drama of the quiet night. Once they were inside the sanctuary, there were specific procedures that patients (and nonpatients) were obliged to carry out, as there were for any god in any place (Caton 1900; Edelstein and Edelstein 1945; Meier 1967; Tomlinson 1983). So the social life that was familiar to patients in the outside world was translated or transferred to a special setting—the worldly familiar was brought within the holy and somewhat unfamiliar. Asclepius did not demand elaborate rituals, but they had to be carried out correctly, in the prescribed manner. Sacrifices had to be offered, according to a person's ability to pay. All manner of things were presented, but money and animals were the most usual offerings. During the preparatory rituals, prayers of supplication for healing were also offered up. The singing of hymns was very important—typical was the paeon, a choral rendering accompanied by the cithara. The priests sometimes gave sermons or orations as a form of education. Perhaps the most significant rituals were those connected with water and purification.

The annual festival at Epidauros was a splendid affair when it was at the height of its popularity. It was celebrated nine days after the festival of Poseidon at Corinth, the Isthmian games, which probably fell toward the end of April. The festival combined religious functions and entertainment and was attended both by ordinary worshipers and Asclepius's representatives from cities all over Greece. In this way, Epidauros showed how it could pull on the strings that tied it to its vast network of sanctuaries. A procession carrying animals for sacrifice and singing paeons of praise made the journey up from Epidauros town and into the hills. Within the sanctuary, there were private and public rites, a banquet, athletic and artistic contests, and plays in the theater.

The pilgrims were kept busy, but when night descended we can imagine a quiet that came, in sharp contrast to the hurly burly of the day. Their minds filled with images of rituals, natural beauty, stimulating conversations, and perhaps the god himself, the patients filed into the abaton where attendants helped them to find resting places for the night. The stage was now set for incubation or dream healing.

Conclusions

The story of dream healing at Epidauros is our first illustration of the themes developed in chapter 1. Although the time and culture are the farthest from the modern world of the three places discussed in this book, I argue that healing environments span space, time, and cultures. Thus it is instructive to examine how the natural, built, symbolic, and social environments of Epidauros contributed to its healing sense of place.

Epidauros lies in a remote area of gently rolling hills where the beauties of nature can be enjoyed in relative tranquility. Water, scarce in Greece and essential to healing in many cultures, was present, as were groves of trees. Furthermore, the healing god Asclepius was associated with the snake and the dog. The built environment of Epidauros consisted of an ecology of sacred buildings, a set of magnificent structures used for both sacred and profane purposes, which blended with the natural world. Buildings such as the temple of Asclepius and the tholos were both awe-inspiring and functional, creating a sense of trust in the healing powers of the god.

Several aspects of the symbolic environment contributed to the reputation of Epidauros. The site was on sacred ground, located lower than Apollo's abode and yet above where most mortals dwelled. Healing was based on dreams that the Greeks (and many other societies) believed to have great symbolic importance to their lives. Adding as well to the symbolic atmosphere were myths about the origins and life of Asclepius that may be interpreted as relating to the opportunities and constraints of medicine. Finally, it has been shown that certain features of the social environment of the place were conducive to healing. Although the state of medical knowledge was primitive compared to what we have today, patients and doctors shared this knowledge and often met on a more equal footing than is common now. Both physicians and lay people could relate to Asclepius, a local and personal god. The sanctuary itself was a social leveler, a place where people of different status could mingle for a time as they pursued an active social life.

It is important to recognize that the four environments interacted with one another to create a synergistic healing sense of place. As examples, both water and building architecture had symbolic power, part of the social life involved conversing in sacred groves, and the myths about Asclepius involved natural objects. Thus, it is not possible to single out environments or particular elements within environments as the most important healing factors, especially because, as we have seen, healing itself has physical, mental, spiritual, emotional, and social components.

CHAPTER THREE

❧

Bath: Healing Mineral Springs

At first glance, Bath may not appear to be a good candidate for a case study of a healing place. The world knows Bath primarily because of its glittering social life during the eighteenth century when it was a premier watering place. Healing, especially physical, would seem to be overshadowed by grand architecture and colorful figures such as Beau Nash. Yet, like Epidauros, Bath has a centuries-old history of attracting those seeking cures. Although critics of eighteenth-century Georgian Bath justifiably ridiculed the health care provided to many, the mineral springs were thought by Celts, Romans, and Georgians alike to be healing. This chapter tells Bath's story, using, again, a framework of four environments. I will show how even the seemingly nonhealth-related features of Bath such as John Wood's building designs and eighteenth-century social customs were important to its reputation as a healing place.

Rugged Beauty and Jehovah's Blessing

In contrast to the gently rolling hills that nestle the Epidaurian sanctuary, the site of Bath inspires by its rugged beauty (Cunliffe 1969, 1986; Gadd 1971; Lees-Milne and Ford 1982). It, too, is surrounded by hills, at the southern end of the Cotswolds, but these are flat-topped hills split by rivers that cut deeply into the oolitic limestone and Jurassic rock. The city is enclosed, like an arena, by steep limestone cliffs. On three sides

43

flows a meander of the River Avon, a river so sluggish that one wonders how it had the energy to carve such a deep valley. The southern part of the original Roman site, around the mineral springs, is low-lying and swampy, but the ground rises toward the north, leading onto well-drained land, and then turns steeply upward into the Lansdown uplands.

Despite its dramatic natural setting, Bath has had its detractors. In the eighteenth century, a description popular among the sophisticated called it "a place standing in a hole; on a quagmire; impenetrable to the very beams of the sun; and so confined by almost inaccessible hills, that people have scarce room to breathe in the town, or to come at it without danger to their lives" (Neale 1973a, 254, quoted from Wood, 1765, preface).

The site appears to have been chosen for settlement, first by Celtic peoples and later by the Romans, for practical reasons. The River Avon is quite easily forded here, and a strategic Roman road, the Fosse Way, which joined the Humber River to Exeter, passed through. However, the place was not suitable for military, market, or administrative functions. From the perspective of the Roman leaders, this was definitely a peripheral location, a far corner of a land they never fully conquered or integrated into their empire (Stewart 1981). The main attraction for the Celts and the Romans, and many others after them, was the mineral waters.

The mineral springs of Bath emerge at several places, but the majority of the water, over 250,000 gallons a day, is found at King's Bath (46 C° or 115 F°), Hot Bath (49 C° or 120 F°), and Cross Bath (40 C° or 104 F°). It has taken thousands of years for the hot mineral water to pass from its source areas in the Mendip and other surrounding hills, through permeable rock, and rise up through fractures and faults in Mesozoic strata of rock (Cunliffe 1986).

To reiterate a point made in the preceding chapter, water is probably the element of the natural environment that is most closely associated in people's minds with healing (Porter 1990). Water is thought to have physiological effects, such as soothing tired muscles or restoring balances among internal fluids; but it also has great symbolic power as we saw in connection with the rites of purification in Epidauros. By the time of the Hippocratic writings, bathing was advocated in Greece for its cleansing and tonic effects. It was used to adjust the four humors by heating, cooling, moistening, or drying. Thermal water, it was believed, could ease aches and pains, promote good breathing, relieve fatigue, cure headaches, and soften the body so that it could assimilate the nutrients in food (Jackson 1990). *Airs, Waters, and Places*, the major work attributed to Hippocrates, also warned against the unhealthy potential of stagnant water and the miasmic fogs arising from swamps.

As we shall see later, Celtic peoples were attracted to the gushing mineral springs. The Romans who built the original baths at Bath were following a well-established classical tradition. Following their departure from Britain, the use of baths for medicinal and social purposes declined, but never disappeared entirely (McIntyre 1981; Mitchell 1986). In Christian England, springs and holy wells continued as religious sites, each one dedicated to a saint and used for cures for specific ailments. The Protestant reformers closed down holy wells, but, beginning in the sixteenth century, Greek and Roman ideas about the efficacy of mineral waters were revived, based on medical rather than religious grounds.

Continental Europe preceded Britain in its enthusiasm for spas—the word spa comes from the Walloon word *espa* or "fountain," and Spa was the name of a Belgian town near Liege. Taking his cue from the continent, William Turner was the first to reintroduce the use of mineral waters in England. In 1562 he published a book on English waters, mentioning only Bath, but a proliferation of treatises on other springs followed, all extolling their curative powers. By the late-seventeenth century many English towns were developing as social centers for the local gentry and the middle classes. These people now had enough disposable income to indulge in pleasurable pursuits, either in earnest or as an excuse, which often centered around health, but included much else besides. The popularity of balneology (the scientific study of bathing and medicinal springs) grew to the extent that the eighteenth century has been called the "age of watering places." Tunbridge Wells, Epsom, Scarborough, and Harrogate are among the best known spas, but there were, in 1740, over two hundred others in England (McIntyre 1981; Mitchell 1986).

With strong competition from such a large number of aspiring spa towns, Bath had to make an effort to see that its baths (as well as other amenities) were of a sufficient standard to attract visitors in substantial numbers. Evidently they fell short in the sixteenth century, as Turner wrote in his 1562 book that, "There is money enough spent on cock-fightings, tennis playing, parties, banquettings, pageants and plays serving for only a short time of pleasure . . . but I have not heard tell that any rich man hath spent upon these noble baths, being so profitable for the whole Commonwealth of England, one groat these twenty-nine years [since the dissolution of the monasteries by Henry VIII]" (Turner quoted in Rolls 1978, 47). The city corporation took note of the lack and proceeded to develop a complex of baths. The Roman baths had been covered over and forgotten for centuries, but springs still existed that could be tapped.

The close alliance of church and state in providing meaning to the waters is captured in this ode above the common pump in the King's Bath:

> Jehovah's Blessing let's admire,
> Here's constant Heat, and yet no Fire;
> Bethesda's Pool, by sacred Hand,
> Hither remov'd to heal the Land.
> God and the King are here our free Imparters,
> God gives the Waters, and the King the Charters.
> (*Bath and Bristol Guide* 1755, 8)

The Builders of Bath

The built environment of Bath reflects a succession of civilizations that rose and fell in this part of England. Flint implements excavated in the hills surrounding Bath indicate that settlement here was quite intensive in the Neolithic and early Bronze Ages (Cunliffe 1986; Gadd 1971; Haddon 1973; Winsor 1980; Wriston 1978). The Celts probably left the mineral springs in their natural state, but they, and succeeding generations, altered the site itself by building dwellings, sacred places, public works, and other constructions. Relatively little was done to alter the landscape, however, until the rural calm of the West Country was shattered in 43 A.D. with the arrival of the Roman army. Although Bath was not a Roman military stronghold or a regional capital, it was an important node in the frontier communication system. The main functions that Bath came to perform were that of a religious center in combination with one of the great medicinal spas of the Roman world.

The first really splendid buildings at Bath were constructed by the Romans (figure 3.1). In a clever and also politically pragmatic move,

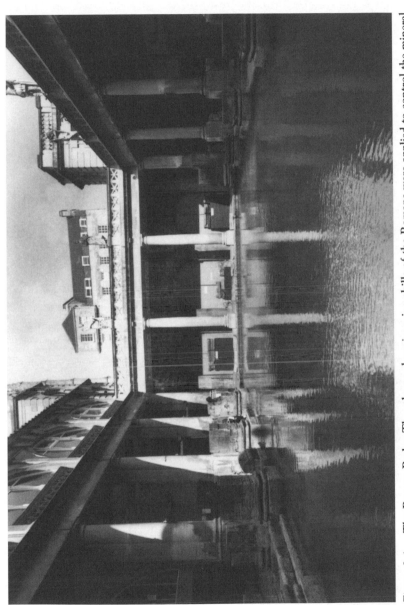

Figure 3.1. The Roman Baths. The advanced engineering skills of the Romans were applied to control the mineral springs and provide rest and recreation. Covered over for centuries, the baths were rediscovered in the late-nineteenth century. Photo courtesy of Lucy Gunning.

the Romans, in the 60s A.D., began to construct a cluster of monumental buildings centered round the temple of Sulis Minerva; the name joined the Celtic goddess Sulis with the Roman Minerva. In both Welsh and old Irish, *Suil* or *Sulis* means an orifice, gap, or eye, making connections to the physical attributes of the site. Also, like Epidauros, the place was in communication with the underworld (Stewart 1981). Temples and baths, godliness and cleanliness, were developed next to each other in an integrated complex that served the triple functions of religious worship, bathing for healing, and social gathering place. The complex included the sanctuary, a classical tetrastyle or four-columned building in the Corinthian order, and a large suite of baths.

The Romans, in contrast to the previous inhabitants, possessed the engineering, plumbing, and building skills necessary to tame the gushing thermal waters. They removed the mud and rubble at the head of the spring, and the fissures through which the thermal waters escaped were enclosed by a watertight wall that was lined inside with lead. The level of technology marshaled to accomplish this engineering feat and to continually flush out the black sand brought up by the spring was remarkable. It is worth noting that one of the dedications at the Cross Bath was to Asclepius—an indication of the healing god's diffusion to the far corners of empire, as well as an affirmation of Bath's healing powers (Cunliffe 1969).

In the early second century A.D., a tholos or ornamental circular temple was added to the complex (reminding us of the tholos at Epidauros, which was also added after the main temple was built) and around 300 A.D. the whole complex was reorganized so that the classical architectural style was replaced with a more native Romano-Celtic style. At this time the open spring was covered with a massive, vaulted, masonry hall that would have added a great deal of mystery to the place.

Following the Roman occupation, the built landscape at Bath went through several phases, but the magnificent buildings that tens of thousands of sight-seers flock to see every year were constructed in the eighteenth century. At the end of the seventeenth century, Bath was still a walled city, but it was ready to burst its seams (Bezzant 1980; Haddon 1973). The satirist Jonathan Swift could say at this time, "Everyone is going to Bath," but the Bath they were going to was in a sorry state. The buildings were dilapidated, there was a wide gap between a wealthy clientele and a poverty-stricken underclass, and the streets were dangerous, filled with ruffians, rapacious sedan-chair men who conveyed clients to the baths, and young gallants who settled disputes with the sword. The anonymous author of *A Step to the Bath* described his feelings about the place in 1700: "During the Season it hath as many Families in a House as *Edenborough*; . . . the *Baths* I can compare to nothing but the *Boylers* in *Fleet-lane* or *Old-Bedlam*, for they have a reeking steem all the year. In a word, 'tis a Valley of Pleasure, yet a sink of Iniquity. Nor is there any Intrigues or Debauch Acted at London, but is mimick'd there" (quoted in Neale 1973b, 39).

Bath entered the eighteenth century as a preindustrial city that was unique in achieving economic success based on providing leisure activities to a ruling elite (Neale 1973a, 1973b). Its leading citizens had taken advantage of an agricultural surplus, the wool trade, and the attractions of the waters to amass several small fortunes. Several noteworthy architects and builders made substantial contributions to the human-made landscape of Bath, but the outstanding figure was John Wood, often referred to as the Elder to distinguish him from his architect son.

Wood was a truly Renaissance person, teaching himself architecture and also astronomy, mythology, and finance. From his reading about the ancient Greek and Roman worlds, he conceived the idea of constructing a New Rome on the site of Bath (Cunliffe 1986). His inspiration for the innovative and beautiful edifices he built was the late Renaissance Italian architect Palladio, who in turn built on the Roman style (Bezzant 1980). Wood's genius was to combine materials found nearby (Bath limestone), Palladian designs, and consistent scale, to produce one of the few cities anywhere that represents an age, Georgian Bath (Haddon 1973).

What Wood, along with his son, created was not easy. He had to accumulate capital, and in order to do that he had to overcome periodic shortages of money, problems with his local labor force, questions of land ownership, and satisfying the nonartistic architectural tastes of his wealthy patrons. At the same time, he was a person who sought to find expression for his own artistic impulses. This set up a creative tension between his artistic and entrepreneurial sides, requiring him to make compromises, which nonetheless produced some of the finest buildings ever designed and constructed (Neale 1973a, 1973b). A case in point is the King's Circus, which he designed and his son built. The building is a masterpiece, but the money came from local Quakers who made their money from the West Indies slave and sugar trades.

Creating Myths, Symbolic Designs, and Healing Rhetoric

There are several reasons to believe that the Celts would have been strongly attracted to the hot springs of Bath. In the pagan world, springs were thought to be places where deities lived and also evidence of the abundance of Mother Earth (Stewart 1981). Water sources were extremely sacred and the creation of life was believed to have taken place in a boiling cauldron. The Celts also had a strong belief in the other world, which was under the ground and was entered through a cave, cavern, well, mysterious opening, or spring. In Celtic myths there are many stories of journeys to and from the other world, a source of both life and death. The chthonic nature of the Celtic gods is clear. It is also fairly clear that the Bath hot springs were a center for Celtic religious worship and ritual, centering on a mother goddess.

The following ode, by T. Watson, seen in the pump room near the Hot Bath, reveals an attempt to link the baths to classical themes and ancient myths:

> "Hygeia" broods with watchful wing
> O'er ancient Badon's mystic spring;
> And speeds from its sulphureous source
> The strong torrent's secret course;
> And fans the eternal sparks of hidden fire
> In deep unfathom'd beds below,
> By Bladud's magic taught to glow;
> Bladud! high theme of Fancy's Gothic lyre.
>   (*Improved Bath Guide* 1825, 42)

The point was made in the preceding chapter that myths, like those surrounding the human/god Asclepius, contribute to the making of places. Bath also has a myth that involves a special person, in this case a king named Bladud, praised in Watson's poem and said by some to be descended from a Trojan prince. Like many myths, Bath's legend has been told in many ways, but the basic story goes something like this (Winsor 1980; Wriston 1978). As a young man, Bladud contracted leprosy and so was banished from the court of his father who was a king in England's West Country. To keep himself, he became a swineherd and infected his pigs with his disease. Then one day the pigs began to wallow in the mud at a spot where the ground never froze and were miraculously cured of their leprosy. Bladud cured himself in the mud and returned home to be welcomed with open arms. He lived to become king and sire a future sovereign, King Lear. There are a couple of embellishments of interest to this basic tale. One says that when he grew old, Bladud became foolish, put on a pair of wings, jumped from a pinnacle of a temple he had built to the goddess Minerva, and perished. It was also said that Bladud traveled to Greece as a young man, about 480 B.C., under the name of Abaris, High Priest of Apollo and spent eleven years there studying with Pythagoras (Neale 1973b).

The date when this story was first told is not known, but it has been repeated many times, first by Geoffrey of Monmouth (d. 1154 A.D.) in his *History of Kings*. John Wood, the foremost eighteenth-century Bath architect, angry at those who scoffed at the Bladud story, put the tale into his essay "Toward a Description of Bath." Although the incidents were supposed to have occurred several centuries B.C., we can infer that those who first related this myth were very familiar with two stories from the New Testament: the one about the man who was cured when his demons were transferred to a herd of swine and the parable Jesus told about the prodigal son. Just as we found Asclepian healing traits to be attributed to Jesus Christ, we find here an attempt to Christianize a pagan myth.

There is, possibly, medical truth in the Bladud legend, but the tale's veracity is not what gives it its enduring force. Myths symbolize what a group of people feels to be important in their relationships to their environment, in their dealings with one another, and the mysterious powers that created the world (Stewart 1981). Therefore, it is evident that, at least by the time of Geoffrey of Monmouth, the healing functions (physical, psychological, and societal) of Bath's waters were uppermost in people's minds. Furthermore, the therapeutic function was allied to religious sentiments that included belief in the miraculous and in supernatural powers. Thus the Bladud story, with its ties to near-supernatural royalty, miraculous cures, and the Bible, helped through the years to symbolize Bath's premier position as a healing place.

The myth is open to further interpretations. It might refer to curing mental illness or to the mending of broken social relationships. The seekers after pleasure who ate too much and drank too much, complained of gout, and sought relief in the baths might have been cheered by the forgiveness granted to the prodigal son. The story about Bladud jumping off a temple, might, like Asclepius's raising the dead and subsequent punishment by the gods, be a cautionary tale against overweening pride.

The Bladud myth arises from British mythology, which in turn is mainly derived from Celtic mythology (Stewart 1981). Celtic deities were closely linked to specific locales. Thus they are analogous to the chthonic nature of Asclepius, in contrast to the more universal nature of the Greek Olympians. Since Celtic religion and mythology were strongly related to the physical environment, it is logical to expect that the Bladud legend is connected to the physical characteristics of the Bath site.

The architect John Wood built his marvels in the eighteenth century, but as we noted earlier his spirit dwelled in a mythical past. Neale (1973a, 1973b) has discovered pre-Roman Celtic, pre-Hellenic Jewish, Greek, and Roman traditions in his work. In order to understand his interpretation or reading of the landscape he was trying to create, one must understand his various writings on architecture and ancient mythologies. He had an idea, wholly unsubstantiated, that Bath was only the core of what once was a city the size of Babylon, built around 480 B.C. by the mythical King Bladud. This fantasy landscape was peopled by Druids, Greeks, and Britons who built temples, castles, and palaces in the antique style. Wood had read in the Hippocratic writings that cities "that face the East, and are sheltered from the Westerly winds, RESEMBLE the SPRING . . . the Inhabitants have good Complexions; and the Women, besides being very fruitful, have easy times" (Wood 1765, 56–57). Bath faced the east and was sheltered from westerly winds and so, Wood said, must resemble the season of spring and be youthful and forever happy.

We spoke earlier of Wood's creative tension between his artistic impulses and his need for capital. He also had to resolve a conflict between his deep Christian faith and his love of pagan antiquity (Neale 1973a, 1973b). In particular, he worried that what he was building was almost entirely secular. To relieve his anxiety, he turned to the use of symbols in his architecture, especially the circle and the square, which he believed were inspired by God, the Divine Architect (figure 3.2). He used these two geometric designs extensively in such masterpieces as the Queen Square (completed in 1734) and the King's Circus (completed by his son in 1758). The central area of Queen Square, for example, features a square and inside it a circle.

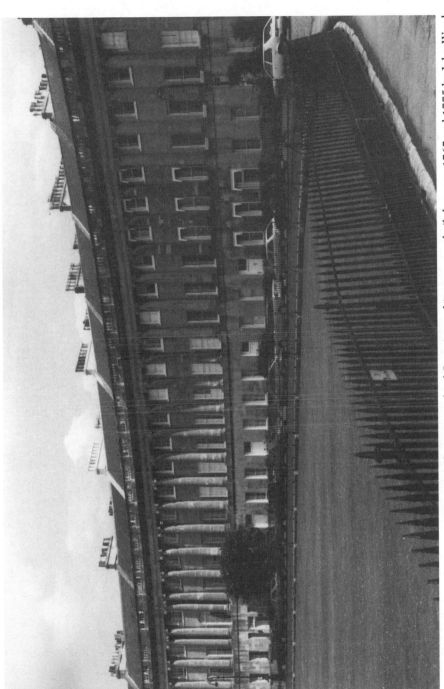

Figure 3.2. The Royal Crescent. This magnificent example of Georgian architecture was built between 1767 and 1775 by John Wood the Younger. Photo courtesy of Lucy Gunning.

The circle, symbolizing perfection and often found in both Celtic and Jewish designs, was preferred by Wood to the square. Several different types of threefold imagery were associated with the circle. The human figure, the image of God, was often decomposed into the head, trunk, and limbs in the thinking of the time. When these three parts of the body were stretched out as in the Vitruvian Figure, they could be encompassed by either the circle or square. The King's Circus is the best example of Wood's use of both the circle and threefold symbolism. Two concentric circles define the outer and inner walls of three sections of buildings. (Is it a coincidence that the outer circle's dimensions correspond to those of the chalk wall at Stonehenge?) One approaches the Circus along three streets. Like the temple complex at Epidauros, the buildings feature the three principal Greek orders of columns, appearing one above the other. On the bottom story is Doric Robust Man, above that is Ionic Grave Matron, and at the top is Corinthian Sprightly Young Girl.

One can usually interpret the use of symbols in different ways. I would suggest that Wood drew his designs and built with a Renaissance view of the world in mind. This perspective had at its core two key ideas: an analogy between the human body and the cosmos or universe and a search for order, manifested in the idea of the Great Chain of Being, which put every object in nature, including humans, in their place (Bamborough 1980; Mills 1982). These concepts led to the following interpretation of the human condition. Order among humans was essential for physical and mental health. But order had been disrupted by the fall from God's grace. The result was drunkenness, uncontrolled passion, and madness. However, one could counteract these disorderly tendencies by constructing works of art and architecture with harmonious, balancing designs such as the circle and square. Thus architecture based on the human body (recall the Vitruvian Figure and the stages of life depicted in the statues that decorate the King's Circus) was designed to bring health to the people. I also speculate that geometric forms are like mandalas, which are thought in many societies to represent healing and wholeness.

Symbolic environments are created in many ways, including the rhetoric used by those who take opposing positions in conflicts. Let us examine the beliefs and language used to support these beliefs in the controversy surrounding the ability of Bath's waters to cure physical illnesses. Doctors, chemists, and others, beginning in the seventeenth century, became very interested in analyzing the spa waters in order to improve their use in treatments, identify impurities that could be removed, and propose similar mixtures as medicines. A major part of the difficulty in assessing the merits of spa water or any type of water, however, was the technical problems involved in the process of analysis (Coley 1982, 1990; Hamlin 1990). When serious experiments began, the state of the art in chemistry was woefully inadequate to make reliable and accurate judgments possible. Analysis was by trial and error and controversial claims were inevitable. A standard technique was to examine the residue left after evaporation, but the materials left were often too minute to detect with current methods, many compounds were similar in composition, and chemical changes may have occurred during the evaporation process. There was still a great deal of skepticism about a science that trailed vestiges of alchemy from the Middle Ages. However, analytical techniques improved and some progress was made, although much of the "scientific" reporting was verbose and polemical, aimed at blinding the public with science. The rise of pneumatic chemistry turned attention away from mineral solids to the contents of various gases in the water, which some saw as the most important curative agents. In fact, the history of progress in inorganic chemistry at this time could be traced through water analysis.

One way of looking at the water efficacy controversy is to contrast the scientific analysis of the waters with the medical evidence of cures (Hamlin 1990; Rolls 1978, 1988). Supporting the medical view in the seventeenth and eighteenth centuries was the idea that the medicinal properties of specific springs were "unique, irreducible, and inimitable." Local waters contained a "spirit" or "life" or "soul" that could not be captured. One had to drink at the place itself to receive full benefit. But chemical evidence, as we have seen, had little to show after centuries of experiments. The elements deemed necessary for cures simply could not be found.

By the nineteenth century the struggle between chemical analysis and medical testimony was being won by chemistry, but the controversy was by no means laid to rest. Today, the argument resembles that between holistic and reductionist medicine. The latter approach, finding nothing of value in Bath water, would deny that Bath was a truly curative place. A holistic perspective would admit the failure of chemical analysis, but would also point to the potential efficacy of a much wider range of environmental and social factors. Here, the uniqueness of a place comes once again to the fore, not in terms of a mysterious "soul" in the waters, but in terms of scenery, diet, and amusements, the whole range of elements that heal both mind and body. In 1897 a physician wrote that the quiet of Bath, fresh air, and long hours of rest, not the waters, would help ladies of fashion who had spent long nights in air polluted by gas lamps.

The story of Dr. George Kersley is one more illustration of the conflict between what science says should happen and what actually is observed in medical practice. Kersley was a physician in the hospital for rheumatic diseases for thirty years. He was very successful in raising rheumatology to a scientific discipline and for getting rid of the connection between Bath water and magic. In so doing, he contributed to the decline of the town as a watering place. However, Kersley experienced a change of heart when he realized that the mineral springs had once been effective because of the placebo effect; that is, people who believed that Bath water could cure, might indeed feel better. He remarked that he and his colleagues had done a disservice by "knocking the spook out of the waters" (Rolls 1988) and became one of the most active advocates of reestablishing Bath as a spa.

The Social Lives of the People of Bath

For the Celts, Bath's mineral waters were a gathering place for religious ritual. For the Romans, too, Bath became a social place. We can imagine groups of middle class Roman citizens from many parts of the Roman Empire coming to the baths to be washed, oiled, sanded, stripped with a bronze stirgil blade, and massaged; to gossip, conduct business, relax, play games, and worship at the temple. Tacitus (c. 55–120) thought he saw an ulterior motive in the Roman construction of a site for rest and recreation. It was, he claimed, a ploy to subdue the warlike Celts and lure them into a soft life. "In this way," he said, "people learnt to mistake the path of servitude for the high road of culture" (Wriston 1978, 9).

When Queen Elizabeth I visited Bath in 1574, she was shocked by the state of the Abbey Church and established a nationwide restoration fund. In 1590 she granted the city a charter of incorporation. The new city authorities were entrepreneurs, anxious to establish the well-being of Bath, and at the same time line their own pockets. Meanwhile, Bath's reputation for care and cure began to attract the destitute in increasing numbers. They were followed, during the sixteenth century, by members of the middle and upper classes, who came in seasonal swarms. Travel was now easier and more secure, and patrons of the baths were influenced by a spate of medieval writings that praised the benefits of bathing. During the sixteenth and seventeenth centuries, Bath depended less on the wool trade and consciously developed its tourist industry. Accommodations for visitors and recreational facilities were built.

A series of visits by members of royal families gave a tremendous boost to the city as royalty set the stamp of approval on a place for the wealthy and fashionable (Cunliffe 1986; Gadd 1971; McIntyre 1981). Queen Elizabeth I came in 1574 and 1591, Ann of Denmark in 1677, and James II with his second wife, Mary of Modena, in 1687. Most important was the coming of Princess Anne, who had gout, in 1688 and 1692, and then return visits in 1702 and 1703 as Queen Anne. These later visits were attended with great ceremony, orchestrated by the city corporation.

Bathing in Georgian times was an elaborate ritual (Lees-Milne and Ford 1982; McIntyre 1981; Rolls 1988). Typically, patrons were fetched early in the morning from their lodgings by sedan-chair men and brought to the baths. They entered "slips" where they undressed and donned attire suitable for the baths. In the seventeenth century some people objected to nude mixed bathing, and by the eighteenth century more decorum was practiced. Fashionable ladies walked into the water with little trays that contained sweetmeats, nosegays, handkerchiefs, and patches attached to their necks by ribbons. Many bathers fell over into the water and had to be helped up by "bath guides." Pumps for dousing the whole body or concentrating on certain spots also became available. Later, drinking the waters rather than bathing in them became popular, recommended more and more by physicians. During the life of the spa many ways of using the waters were tried, including immersion, spraying or douching in all of the body's orifices, drinking the water hot or cold, mixing water with mud, mixing in pine and sulfur and cardamoms, sitting in a sweating box, and passing electric shocks through the water.

All the baths were uncovered and crowds watched the spectacle from the galleries. There was clearly much scope here for comedy and no doubt the onlookers made jeering remarks; in an age of satire, the bathing behavior of the rich and pseudo-rich was an obvious target for the barbs of wits. The most famous satirical commentary is Anstey's *The New Bath Guide: Or, Memoirs of the B-r-d Family* (1767), which purported to be the letters written home by various members of a family somewhat out of their social depth in Bath. One of the characters writes: "And to-day many persons of rank and condition / Were boil'd by command of an able physician" (44). Thomas Rowlandson, social satirist and caricaturist, made a series of drawings that he called "Comforts of Bath." One shows men and women plunging about together under the bewildered gaze of King Bladud. They are gasping from the shock of the hot water, some cling to columns, all are wearing day clothes; they are not of the highest social order (Lees-Milne and Ford 1982).

Do people make the times or do the times make people? Some would argue that three men, Richard "Beau" Nash, John Wood, and Ralph Allen, were largely responsible for creating eighteenth-century Bath, but the reverse is probably more true. Bath had created an environment in which people with their talents could be shown to great advantage (Neale 1973a). Wood the architect was blessed with a growing demand for housing development, Allen's financial genius suited a mostly booming economy, and Nash was able to take advantage of a clientele that craved both order and frivolity. For our purposes, it is sufficient to talk about only two of these men in detail. We have already discussed Wood's creation of a highly symbolic architectural environment. Now we turn to Nash for his influence on the social environment.

When Nash arrived he found a town that was dangerous, chaotic, and filled with ruffians and rapacious sedan-chair men (who transported people around the town), a place where quarrels were settled openly with the sword. Realizing that these conditions would have to change if the city were to attract the wealthy ill and the gamblers of London, Nash, backed by the city corporation, moved in various ways to alter the social environment radically (Austen-Leigh 1939; Bezzant 1980; Gadd 1971; Haddon 1973; Lees-Milne and Ford 1982; Sitwell 1987). Nash may have been superficial and trivial in many ways, but he had a passion for order and propriety that the genteel appreciated. He regulated lodging fees, improved the roads, kept the streets clean, forbade the wearing of swords, and stopped the street fighting. To put an end to the intimidating behavior of sedan-chair men, only the sixty licensed by the city were allowed to operate. Fees were set according to the distance they carried people.

The Bath and Bristol Guide (1755) provided several pages of exact yardage between important points throughout the city, and fines were imposed for overcharging or insulting passengers.

Nash's rules dictated the daily life of people taking the waters. Here is a schedule for the day: serious health seekers to attend the baths from 6 to 9 in the morning; breakfast in lodgings or Assembly Rooms until 10:30; drink the waters or watch late bathers until 12; morning service in the Abbey at noon; walking, riding, shopping, and reading until 2:30; dinner and parading until tea at 5 in the Assembly Rooms; visits, gaming, dancing, and theater until 11 at night when everything promptly ceased. Even the highest born could not escape the daily schedule. It is said that Nash refused to grant permission to Princess Amelia to dance beyond the proscribed closing hour. The rules seem petty, but they served a purpose. They were not intended to keep people of fashion in line, as they knew the rules and kept them instinctively; rather, they were for those who aspired to fashion, did not know the rules, and needed to be reined in.

The effect of all the rules was to create a society with civilized manners that diffused throughout England. Nash was famous for calling down people who were snobbish to people of a lower class (the working classes excepted). He frowned on private parties that encouraged cliquishness and forced people to meet and mix at places like the Assembly Rooms and the theater. Thus, in contrast to London, where social distinctions remained sharp, Bath, at least on the surface and above a certain class, developed an open society. However, the skeptical novelist Tobias Smollett remarked that this rather spurious social leveling was a sort of forgetfulness about social relations, as if the hot springs were the River Lethe.

As we have seen, controversies over water efficacy were often clouded by underlying quarrels that were far more political and social than they were medical or chemical. Another contentious issue involved legitimization for spas and doctors (Coley 1990; Hamlin 1990; Harley 1990). Before the seventeenth century, legitimization was based on religious grounds, but as scientific knowledge developed, physicians and spa entrepreneurs sought the legitimacy that science was beginning to offer. A Protestant physician, Walter Bailey, said in 1587 that water use should be supervised by scientists, rather than priests, because God provided water as a natural, not a supernatural means of healing. Chemical analysis of the water in itself helped to legitimize spa practices, despite the fact that results were contradictory and that there were fundamental divisions concerning appropriate theory and practice among chemists. Science then, as now, was coopted to add authority to curative claims.

Although spas usually achieve initial success because they attract seekers after health, they also attract those who wish to exploit them for commercial gain. Both physicians and entrepreneurs recognized Bath's potential for enormous profits (Rees 1985). One advertising ploy was to create an image of mystery or magic around the mineral springs. No one really understood how, or even if, the water could cure, but many people were willing to believe that a certain something, a spirit perhaps, dwelled in the springs. Bath also benefited from an image of being radical or out of the mainstream because it was touted as an alternative to the mainstream medicine of the day. At the same time, it was presented as a respectable place. This last image was bolstered by reference to its continental origins, by the use of medical language in describing cures, and by recommendations from physicians themselves.

Attempts at legitimacy were contested, primarily by doctors, and often by those who were outside the spa establishment. Physicians at Bath and other spas were assailed by people who questioned their claims and authority (Coley 1982; Neve 1984; Rolls 1978). Several issues became symbolic focal points for essentially political economic debates. One was the question of whether Bath waters had special properties or whether ordinary tap water would do just as well. Bath insiders, as we have seen, made many special, if changing, claims for efficacy, but outsiders such as Smollett begged to differ.

It must be remembered that physicians in eighteenth-century Britain, as in ancient Greece, held a far lower status than they do in the Western world today. Not surprisingly, Bath attracted its share of imposters and quacks, willing to cash in on a good thing. A gullible public could be told by fraudulent physicians that they had a wide range of ailments and then be sold all kinds of treatments for them (Schnorrenberg 1984). Dame Edith Sitwell, in a fictionalized account of Beau Nash, wrote satirically of these charlatans: "(He) . . . perceived that the cloud he had taken for a universe of ravens, or for locusts, was, in fact, a cloud of quack-doctors who had gathered together to pursue the invalids to the Baths" (1987, 25–26).

The Lessons of Bath

At the close of the preceding chapter, I began a process of drawing out some threads of meaning from the stories of three healing places. I want to continue that process now with Bath, using the same four environments as framework and amplifying them with the material from this chapter. We first look at the *natural environment* or physical setting. Bath's steep hills and rambling river make a strong contrast to the gentle slopes and overall dryness of Epidauros, but the natural environment is nonetheless appealing to many visitors. Here, the main focus from Celtic times to the present has been on the tremendous outpourings of hot mineral water from the springs. Again, we emphasized that water was the element most associated with healing. At Bath, the water had both its sacred uses (by the Celts in ancient times) and secular uses (by the Romans and Georgians). Most notably, Bath became the most prestigious English spa, for a time during the eighteenth century, as church and state converged to sanction the mineral springs. Another important feature of Bath's physical environment was, like Epidauros, remoteness or distance from major population centers. It was on the fringes of Roman Britain, and even in the eighteenth century was only accessible by the landed gentry or nouveau riche.

Turning to the *built environment*, we see that still another similarity between Epidauros and Bath is the extraordinary architecture, the finest examples of their place and time. In particular, we praised the massive Roman baths and the Sulis Minerva temple complex and of course the eighteenth-century splendors designed and built by John Wood and son. Roman building was characterized by spectacular feats of engineering that channeled the waters into useful places for rest and recreation. Following a period of decline in building after the Romans departed, a new entrepreneurial age based on a booming local economy spawned a new spate of building by Wood and others. What the built environment contributed to Bath's reputation as a healing place, at least in Roman and Georgian times, was a sense of grandeur and power, what Yi-fu Tuan (1974) would characterize as public symbols.

Many aspects of Bath could be singled out as contributing to its *symbolic environment*; four were chosen here. First was Celtic beliefs and rituals connected with the underworld that figured prominently in their mythology. The central myth at Bath is the story of King Bladud, certainly not a well-known name today, but nonetheless one that was familiar at the time of the Georgians. Most important is the healing connotations of the myth, both in physical and social terms. Then there was the complex symbolism of John Wood's designs that reflected a diverse collection of ancient mythologies. Once more, these symbols can be connected to health and wholeness. Finally, the ideologies and language expressed in debates over the ability of the mineral springs to cure physical ailments contributed another element to the symbolic environment.

Throughout the centuries, people came to Bath to be cured physically, but they were also attracted by the *social environment*. It is my claim that the activities people engaged in at places such as Epidauros and Bath contributed to a sense of well-being (they might also detract from it if indulged in to excess or improperly). Bath was an important place for rest and recreation for the Romans, and in the eighteenth century it set the standard for proper social conduct for all of Britain. Bathing rituals and Beau Nash's rules created a distinct social milieu. Whether or not there was really social leveling in Georgian Bath, at least many of the lower (not the lowest) social orders felt free to mingle with the upper classes. Another aspect of social conditions in Bath parallels that of Epidauros; in both places physicians and patients were on more of an equal footing than is true today in Western society.

Now that the stories of two healing places have been told, I would like to suggest two more ideas that were not explicitly developed within chapter sections, but which are important nonetheless. Both themes involve paradoxes. First, it must have been noticed that all is not sweetness and light in places such as Epidauros and Bath. In other words, we encountered *conflict*. We know relatively little about controversies in Epidauros, although, as examples, we do know that "scientific" and "divine" medicine clashed at times, and many people thought that the whole idea of dream healings was a fraud. The story of Bath is rife with conflicts over its natural beauty, vice and virtue, pagan and Christian symbolism, historical preservation, water efficacy, what to do with the poor, the legitimacy of physicians, and hygiene. The question is how can a place gain a healing reputation when conflicts abound?

Second, we see from our first two examples that every healing place is unique. That is, the potential for healing may arise in very different circumstances, in different times and places. We can see this easily if we contrast Epidauros with Bath or even Bath with itself in different periods during its evolution. I try to make the case, however, that one can look for common themes that are meaningful, albeit in different ways, in any healing place. I will deal with this *uniqueness/generality* idea again in the Lourdes chapter. I view it as a kind of *metaidea* because it helps to show how the four environments can be applied to current medical situations.

CHAPTER FOUR

❧

Lourdes: Healing Pilgrimages

In 1858, in the village of Lourdes in France, Bernadette, a peasant girl of fourteen, reported seeing apparitions of the Virgin Mary in a grotto beside a river. She reported Mary's messages to the crowds that began to gather. When stories circulated that water from a spring that emerged from the grotto could cure, the reputation of Lourdes as a healing place began. Today, millions come here as pilgrims each year. The religious element is, of course, a powerful and probably the most significant feature in the reputation of Lourdes as a healing place. People obviously come here for spiritual healing, but many, believing in miracle cures, come for physical healing as well. In the summer of 1994, I joined a group of pilgrims on a five-day tour to Lourdes (run by an agency that sponsored visits to Catholic sacred sites) in order to experience firsthand what went on in this famous town. From that experience, I realized that people came for emotional as well as social healing.

Of the three case studies discussed in this book, Lourdes is the only one whose reputation for healing is still current. Applying the four environments to this place shows that the ideas of this book do not only apply to the past. In addition, I hope that relating some of my experiences at Lourdes will add to a sense of immediacy.

A Healing Spring in the Pocket of the Pyrenees

The natural setting of Lourdes, to this observer at least, is the most striking of the three places described in this book. The background, seen not
far in the distance from the town, is the Pyrenees. Located in southwestern France, Lourdes lies at the foot of the spectacular mountain range
that helps to form the border between France and Spain. The town lies
within a rural, agricultural area. Tourists can take day trips into the Pyrenees, where splendid scenic vistas appear around every turn of the road.
The physical geography of the town itself resembles that of Bath, con-
sisting of a group of steep hills rising away from a central river, the Gave.
Not surprisingly, people who truly believe in the apparitions of the Virgin
are inspired by the physical setting. Thus Ruth Cranston writes:

> There it lies, a shining jewel of a town, slipped into the pocket of the
> Pyrenees—spires, towers, green trees and gleaming gardens, dazzling in
> the brilliant southern sunlight. Smiling country—lush fields, flashing
> streams; crisp clear air, resounding all day with the songs of pilgrims, the
> tramp of hurrying feet. (1955, 22)

The example of Bath, once described as a "quagmire," reminds us that
not everyone can see the beauty of a healing place. One visitor to Lourdes,
Daniel Barbe, who came there toward the end of the nineteenth century,
called Lourdes "one of the most obscure and lowly of the towns of France"
(Barbe 1894, 3) and said that the traveler was disappointed as he ap-
proached the town because there was nothing particularly charming to be
seen. However, he also felt obliged to report being impressed with the River
Gave and the churches that were the architectural focus of his pilgrimage.

Recall that Epidauros lies in a remote spot and that Bath, at least in
Celtic and Roman times, was at the periphery of human activity. Although there are exceptions, a common feature of pilgrimage sites associated with many religions is that they, too, are often located in areas that
are relatively isolated or far from concentrations of human populations.
Travel to such a site enables pilgrims to get away from the stresses of
everyday life for a time. Lourdes, despite its millions of annual visitors, is
an isolated place, at the periphery of population centers and human activities. Whether the traveler arrives by walking, bicycle, car, bus, or
plane, one must make a substantial effort to get there.

It is interesting to learn that Lourdes is not the only place in this rather remote corner of France where the Virgin Mary is reported to have appeared. Indeed, one can map out a total of ten shrines in what Neame (1968) calls the "Marian Terrain" of the Pyrenees, all of which at one time over the past several centuries attracted a pilgrimage. The shrines form a rough circle within the Catholic dioceses of Tarbes and Bayonne, with the premier site, Lourdes, in the middle—a symbolic geometry of sacred places.

Bernadette never said that Mary talked to her about healing or cures and Bernadette herself suffered illness throughout her entire life. Despite this, Lourdes is known primarily as a healing place. How did this come about? Water, important in both Epidauros and Bath, once again is the key. One thing Mary did say to Bernadette was that the young girl should dig in the dirt on the grotto floor. Bernadette dug and uncovered a trickle of water that later turned into a flowing spring that now produces 30,000 gallons of water a day (Cranston 1955). Within a few days, a story was going around that a blind man had washed his eyes in the spring and recovered his sight. Then people began to talk about a woman whose dying child had recovered after it had been dipped into the water. The crowds that gathered because of Bernadette's reports of apparitions now came to witness healing or be healed.

As we noted in the preceding chapters, it is widely believed that water cleanses, purifies, and heals (Parker 1983). Henri Nouwen, a pilgrim to Lourdes, writes:

> At the grotto, everything speaks of water: the rushing Gave River, the drizzling rain from the cloudy sky, the spring of Masabielle . . . I want to be purified. I want to be cleansed. (1990, 8)

Belief in the power of healing springs is not unusual. Claims have been made for the curative properties of many thermal springs in the Pyrenees, for example, and people in places like Bath made fortunes from selling water cures. There were entrepreneurs at Lourdes who also wanted to capitalize on Bernadette's divinely provided discovery, so they had the water analyzed for its chemical content, hoping to find that elements associated with treatments for specific diseases could be found. Local church and civil authorities, however, also had a hand in the analysis. As

it turned out, there were conflicting reports about the chemical composition of the grotto spring water. The analysis that found no curative elements at all was officially accepted. The implication was that the healing
power of the water had to come from supernatural sources. The entrepreneurs were thus foiled and religion claimed a victory.

Sacred and Profane Built Environments

Many recent visitors to Lourdes must come away thinking, like Barbe,
that much of the town is not particularly charming. Despite the Pyrenees,
the river, and the rugged topography, most of the built environment consists of a crowded conglomeration of hotels, restaurants, and souvenir
shops that cater to the pilgrim and tourist trade. The only place that
Bernadette would recognize, Neame (1968) said, is the grotto, but its pastoral setting and charm are long gone; this is still the case today. There is
little to distinguish the kitschy tourist aspect of the town from any other
place that attracts holiday-makers seeking a good time. What is different
about Lourdes is that there is, literally, another side of town that has a
completely different feel about it; this is the Domain (Rinschede
1986–87).

The Domain of Our Lady contains the grotto where Bernadette reported seeing Mary, as well as the healing spring, baths for women and
men, a three-story basilica, the subterranean Basilica of Pius X, a large
open area for processions, hospitals, and administrative buildings. It is
separated from the rest of the town by fences and gates, but the gates are
usually open and traffic on foot or in wheelchairs passes through quite
freely twenty-four hours a day. The structures in the Domain are, archi-
tecturally speaking, not particularly striking; no John Wood worked here.
They are massive, built to serve large populations of pilgrims. The river is
confined within stone banks as it rushes through, its water still cold from
the mountains.

Rahtz and Watts see Lourdes as "a strange mixture of extreme commercial vulgarity and devout Christian pilgrimage and devotion" (1986,
52). However, I think that the contrast between the Domain and the
"summer town" is symbolically important. One is sacred space; the other
profane (Eliade 1959). The pilgrim or tourist passes quickly between
realms of piety and pleasure, of religious worship and the activities of

daily life. Perhaps it is the sense of hearing that is most affected by the contrast. Coming from profane space through a gate one leaves bustle and noise behind and, the farther one goes within the Domain, the quieter it becomes until there is a hushed silence at the core, the grotto. Imagine sitting up past midnight as I did with a group of pilgrim friends in a bar where loud music is playing, watching raucous crowds of merry-makers pass by, and then sitting a few minutes later with one or two of those friends in meditative silence outside the grotto where the only sounds are the ripple of the river and an occasional whispered voice.

Symbolic Conflicts, Faith, and Journeys

Over the centuries, hundreds of religious pilgrimage sites have been established, flourished for a time, and then faded away. Some, including those dedicated to Mary, have developed a worldwide reputation— Lourdes, Fatima in Portugal, and Guadeloupe in Mexico, for example. What gives sites like Lourdes such staying power, such a strong sense of place? In the previous chapter, there was a discussion of the symbolic rhetoric that arose out of conflicts over the efficacy of the mineral springs at Bath. I suggest that a major factor behind the healing reputation of Lourdes was that it became a symbol for one side in a series of struggles that were taking place in nineteenth-century France.

Bernadette was born into a world that had recently witnessed the tremendous upheavals of the French Revolution and the Napoleonic Wars. Europe was undergoing monumental political, economic, and social upheavals and factions flying the banners of opposing ideologies were vying for power. Napoleon's empire-building ventures had eventually failed; the legacy was political chaos. Meanwhile, the Industrial Revolution had taken hold and bureaucratic institutions were expanding. Many were appalled by what the English poet William Blake called the "Dark Satanic Mills" of the factory system; while others traced the ills of modern Europe to the failure of rationalism. Some of those who reacted to modern lifestyles sought salvation in something beyond earthly things.

As the Nolans (1989) have noted, turning points in European history seem to be connected to the establishment of pilgrimage cults. For example, the Children's Crusades, which took place during the Middle Ages, can be seen as a reaction to deplorable social conditions among the European peasantry. Now, in the mid-nineteenth century, Europe was ripe for Marian pilgrimage (Turner and Turner 1978). Times were particularly bad in the 1850s for the area around Lourdes. There was a severe famine that followed the terrible winter of 1855 and food prices soared over the next couple of years. Peasants rioted at Tarbes, the provincial capital, which is only twelve miles from Lourdes; the emperor sent in his troops to restore order (Neame 1968). This was the political and economic background to Bernadette's report of apparitions in 1858. Although she was a simple peasant girl, she could not help but know what was going on around her. The words that Mary reported fell on the ears of people longing to be free of earthly cares.

As crowds began to come to the grotto for physical and spiritual healing, another disaster struck France. In 1870, Prince Otto Fürst von Bismarck-Schönhausen sent his troops into the country, setting the stage for a vicious struggle between radical and conservative factions within the country. An incident that occurred during this conflict proved to be a turning point for the reputation of Lourdes. A group of pilgrims returning from the town were roughed up at the railway station in Nantes by a group of anti-Catholics. This attack impelled 20,000 pilgrims to travel to Lourdes in 1872 in response. Thus obscure and lowly Lourdes became a symbol for those who supported the Catholic Church against its detractors.

Another dimension of struggle in which Lourdes took sides involved a contest between those who advocated rational, scientific thinking and those who believed in the supernatural and miracles. This was another variation on rational versus irrational thought, which played itself out in Epidauros over two millennia before. As the nineteenth century came to a close, the clergy at Lourdes became more militantly antirationalist. Monseigneur Mermillad, speaking for believers at the consecration of the Basilica at Lourdes in 1876, said:

> Our Lady of Lourdes treads under her feet the double error of our times which seeks to strip the Christian religion of the supernatural and to banish that religion from the social order into the secret place of the individual conscience. (quoted in Barbe 1984, 81–82)

Sometimes a piece of writing brings the opposing sides of a conflict into clear focus while it also heightens emotional exchanges. Such was the case with the novel, *Lourdes*, by the realist, anticlerical writer Emile Zola. The protagonist in the book is a priest who loses his faith and is converted to thinking along scientific lines. Ironically, those who reviled the book usually failed to see that Zola also criticized nineteenth-century medicine; many people went to Lourdes because the medicine available at the time had failed them.

What really happens at Lourdes? Many people have tried to reply to this question; the only thing that can be said for certain about its answer is that it is a contested one. Some put their faith in science and believe that there are scientific explanations for "miracle" cures. But only around sixty-five cures have been authenticated since the Medical Bureau was set up in Lourdes in 1885 to test claims using strictly scientific evidence. What about the rest? True believers have a ready answer. Cures, they say, are effected by supernatural means, perhaps through the intervention of Mary; no other explanation is possible. Skeptics might counter that the whole Lourdes phenomenon is a gigantic hoax; but if it is, it has been carried off extremely well for a long time.

In 1883, the physician Jean-Martin Charcot proposed what he thought was the answer: communal autosuggestion. This was what brought about apparent miracles, he said: people became totally wrapped up in the whole process of preparing for and going on a journey, participating in many hours of rituals, and losing sleep, so that they succumbed to the beliefs and feelings of fellow pilgrims and might thereby be cured of such things as paralysis or certain lesions and tumors (Pope 1989). In other words, Charcot stressed the psychological aspect of healing and based his ideas on the intensity of the religious atmosphere that we noted above. However, he could not explain such claims as the instantaneous mending of broken bones.

The most fundamental reason, I think, for reports of cures at Lourdes, real or imagined, has to do with religious faith. It is hard to think of a symbolic environment more powerful than that which religion provides. Historically, belief in miracles has often been an aspect of faith in many religions (Ranger 1982). Authorities of the Christian Church in the Middle Ages showed their followers miracles in order to instill faith, believing that people had to be shown the concrete actions of God, carried out in their daily lives (Sumption 1975; Thomas 1971). Taking this view of things, one could say that Lourdes became the greatest faith-healing center in the world (Pope 1989).

We saw in the story of Epidauros that the ancient Greeks did not draw a sharp line between what we think of today as rational or irrational thought; nor did they distinguish clearly between divine and earthly causes for such things as cures. The situation has not changed all that much for a large part of the world's population today. Europeans did not clearly differentiate between medicine and magic or science and religion until fairly recently (Pope 1989). Many people continue to believe in miracles; they like the drama involved in the ritual acting out of cures (Thomas 1971). Biomedicine, which has become a dominant paradigm in the twentieth century, has clearly not eliminated such beliefs; witness Lourdes and many other healing sites that are still thriving today.

One cannot simply say that there has been an uninterrupted evolution or transition from magic to medicine, from belief in miracles to rejection of such beliefs (Ranger 1982). There are many Pentecostal Christians, Protestant and Catholic alike, who are true believers in divine interventions in earthly affairs. Even those who are not true believers have to admit that there are still phenomena that lack scientific explanations. We still reserve the term "miracle" for those things we cannot comprehend.

Pilgrimages or journeys from one's home place to holy places have been a common feature in many of the world's religions. Hindus travel to bathe in their sacred rivers, Muslims journey to Mecca, Shintos seek a view of Mt. Fujiyama. European Christian pilgrimage has a long tradition, stretching back several centuries. Some parts of Europe seem to have been more strongly affected by religious movements than others; southwestern France (where Lourdes is located), for example, provided more than its share of pilgrims in the eleventh century. In medieval times, pilgrims often went to holy sites to expiate sin (Sumption 1975). Common people in those days perceived evil, sin, death, and hell as far more real than we do today, and they were willing to make great sacrifices to travel to places where they might be able to rid themselves of these horrors. Many pilgrims came from small, isolated places and wished to confess their sins away from prying eyes and ears in their local communities.

A common belief in medieval Europe was that physical disease had spiritual causes such as sin and so many went on pilgrimages to seek cures. The connection between sin and disease is still prevalent today: witness the contention of many people that AIDS is God's punishment for sexual misdeeds. Turner and Turner (1978, 11) include journeys to expiate disease and sin in what they call "rituals of affliction." That is, the pilgrim undergoes the hardships of a journey, such as exposure to natural hazards, thieves, and even disease itself in order to receive the reward of release from disease and sin at the end.

A pilgrimage always has a specific destination, a sacred place where believers feel that the supernatural has somehow broken through and made contact with the earth (Marnham 1980, Pope 1989). At these places, pilgrims find objects such as statues or relics of a saint and they engage in familiar activities. A chosen few can make religious journeys in the mind to renew their faith or free themselves from sin. Religious authorities recognize, however, that the laity must be encouraged to go on pilgrimages along real roads and be exposed to concrete objects and events.

A typical Catholic pilgrimage begins with a humble person witnessing an apparition of a saint, martyrdom, or a miracle performed by a saint. Only a few may be attracted to the site at first. Then, if a substantial number of people are impressed, say, by promises of miraculous cures, crowds begin to gather (Turner and Turner 1978). The drawing power of particular places changes over time, however, and sites compete with others for visitors (Sumption 1975). Sites also operate at different geographical scales, many achieve only local fame, others attract pilgrims regionally or nationally, still others, like Lourdes, are known worldwide.

I wish to make the argument here that pilgrimage creates a symbolic landscape at a sacred site. That is, in places such as Lourdes, both concrete and abstract symbols provide a variety of significant meanings for believers. There are two ideas about how this comes about. One is that a sacred destination is a "social construction" (one might also say a "cultural construction") in that a variety of actors, including church authorities, entrepreneurs, and pilgrims create out of their beliefs, intentions, and goals in life, such ideas as expiation from sin and divinely sanctioned space and such concrete objects as the relics of saints and holy water that concentrate symbolic meaning in one particular spot.

A second idea is that pilgrimage provides for a symbolic transformation in people's lives. Victor and Edith Turner (1978), borrowing from the work of Arnold van Gennep, describe religious pilgrimage in terms of a rite of passage that goes through three stages. First, at the point of origin, the pilgrim is separated from a familiar, stable set of social relationships. Along the road to the holy site, the traveler is in a "liminal" state, without clear direction, neither one place nor another. Then, once the destination is reached, the pilgrim forms new relationships among others who are true believers. A transformation takes place, and the pilgrim is renewed physically, mentally, and spiritually. I witnessed this transformation in at least one member of my pilgrim group, which I explain later.

Communitas, Intercession, and Bearing Witness

On the surface, life at Lourdes appears to resemble life at a summer resort—crowds of people amble freely around the streets, visiting the shrines and shops in an almost random way. A visitor soon understands, however, that a tremendous amount of organization has taken place, especially in the Domain of Our Lady. One might say that there were attempts at crowd control here from the very beginning. When people hoping to witness miraculous cures first appeared in large numbers at the grotto, local authorities put up barricades to keep them away, but this was futile.

Fourteen years after Bernadette's apparitions, in 1872, the first National Pilgrimage was organized, in large measure as a response to attacks by the French government on the Church. In 1884, the Association of the Hospitallers of Our Lady of Lourdes was established; its task was to transport and care for the sick, as well as to police daily activities. Now, more than four million people come to Lourdes each year. Many of them experience a strong sense of what the Turners (1978) call *communitas* or a group feeling of spiritual renewal. But communitas would hardly be possible without organization.

Not everyone comes to Lourdes seeking communitas, however. Some are tourists who simply want to see what the place is all about. Many come to have a good time, as evidenced by the noisy parties that go on until late at night in the bars and restaurants and out into the streets. Then there are those who make their living from catering to the pilgrim and tourist trade: tour organizers, shopkeepers, and church officials from priests to bishops. Eade (1992), who spent time as a helper in Lourdes, finds that all is not harmony and mutual goodwill in the little world of the town. Rather, he finds groups in conflict, as well as dissonance and ambiguity in social relationships.

Despite underlying tensions, things seem to run smoothly enough from the point of view of an ordinary pilgrim. This seems to me to be based on an unobtrusive and yet firm handling of much of what goes on in the town, reminding one of Beau Nash's rules at Bath. Our group, like children in a summer camp whom their leader wants to run tired, was kept moving almost every hour of the day, from early morning to late evening. There were daily Masses, meals at set times, both an afternoon procession for blessing the sick and an evening candlelight parade, and over forty special places to visit, mostly connected with Bernadette's life and visions. What struck me most forcefully was the way a team of young people, dressed like scouts, standing in strategic places, managed to handle the movement of thousands of marchers in the processions, forming them into lines and directing them to certain places at specific points in the ceremony. One could move around, but only within very definitely set limits.

A very important aspect of the social healing environment at Lourdes is that it enhances a Roman Catholic tradition of putting the common person in touch with God through two intermediaries, Mary and Bernadette. Lourdes is a relatively recent example of a traditional Marian pilgrimage that began in Europe in the twelfth century. Devotion to Mary, like Asclepius's sanctuaries, tended to be very localized; that is, people came to her over rather small distances and associated her with particular places (e.g., Our Lady of Chartres). Sumption expresses this well when he says, "the process by which the veneration of the saints became associated with particular places is especially striking in the case of the Virgin Mary" (1975, 49). And her association with Lourdes is captured when Paignon writes: "Lourdes holds only two people: Our Lady and the childlike collective person who is all the pilgrims" (1956, 162).

Mary has always been very popular among the masses of Catholic faithful. Those who were powerless, weak, or starving believed that she would stand up for them and alleviate their suffering. As we saw in the case of both Bath and Epidauros, myths become a part of the whole atmosphere created in healing places. Similarly, myths or stories are told of Mary's power to overcome the powers of evil and thereby help the helpless. In the Middle Ages, the most popular tale was about a servant named Theophilus who sold his soul to the devil so that he could become the master himself. Although he achieved his aim, he suffered remorse and prayed to Mary for aid. And, even though he had clearly sinned, she seized the contract from Satan and saved the former servant from hell (Sumption 1975).

"At Lourdes, the modern motto is, 'Per Mariam, ad Jesus' (Through Mary to Jesus)" (Meier 1967, 135). This motto expresses the emphasis in recent Marian pilgrimage on Mary as intercessor or intermediary between humans and God. Intercession is a basic tenet of the Catholic faith, an aspect of the doctrine of the Communion of Saints, which joins together the faithful on earth, souls in purgatory, and saints in heaven (Turner and Turner 1978). The doctrine allows for humans to make contact with the divine through a saint. For the common person who feels far removed from God and yet sees someone like Mary as almost like a family member, the attraction of the possibility of intercession is clear.

If Mary provides an accessible link to God or Jesus, then Bernadette, an ordinary peasant girl, provided a link to Mary. Put another way, the belief that Mary appeared and talked to Bernadette represents the Blessed Virgin reaching down to help the downtrodden. Apparitions of Mary are generally witnessed by very ordinary people such as the six teenagers at Medjugorje in the former Yugoslavia and Nancy Fowler in Conyers, Georgia.

Bernadette was born in 1844 in Lourdes. Her father, a mill hand, appears to have been rather feckless and had great difficulty making ends meet for his poor family. She was often ill as a child; when she was eleven she had cholera and she was constantly afflicted with asthma. She was a poor student in the local school and was not even particularly religious until she encountered Mary at the age of fourteen. In other words, she typified the underclass of her day, barely surviving under harsh environmental and social conditions (Marnham 1980; Neame 1968). The Catholic Church eventually made much of Bernadette's appeal to the poor. Here, for example, are the words of M. Mermillad: "Does it not seem as though our God were communicating with us through His poor" (quoted in Barbe 1894, 82). In the same vein, Cranston says, "From having been at first an obscure stepchild, regarded with some hesitation and embarrassment, Lourdes has come to be a beloved daughter; next to Rome, the brightest jewel in the Catholic crown" (1955, 105). Here we have an excellent example of an "underclass" place being elevated and saved from obscurity.

As is the case with so many venerated religious figures, it is difficult at a remove in time to sort out fiction from fact concerning the life and character of Bernadette. What we have said so far appears to be true. We

also know that two years after her apparitions, in 1860, she entered a local convent and became a nun. From 1866 to the end of her life in 1879,
following a prolonged illness, she lived in a convent in Nevers. She was
canonized a saint in 1933 (Turner and Turner 1978).

Much of what is said and believed about Bernadette today is a collection of anecdotes, which Zimdars-Swartz (1991) calls a "selective hagiog-
raphy." These stories of Bernadette's harsh life both emphasize and ro-
manticize it. The qualities imputed to her help common people to see her
as one of them and yet, at the same time, somehow closer to God. One is
reminded of Asclepius here, a bridge between earth and heaven. Stories
are told of her modesty, sincerity, warmth, humbleness, piety, and sense of
humor. When grilled by the authorities, she reported what she saw and
she stuck to her story. Despite her almost unbearably harsh upbringing,
her simple faith shone through to inspire fellow sufferers.

Part of Bernadette's role as intercessor to Mary was to impart to the
faithful what Mary told her during the eighteen apparitions she witnessed. What did Mary say? She asked for three things: unceasing prayer,
processions to the grotto, and that a chapel be built. That is, she called a
world of sinners to repent and renew their faith through rituals and concrete signs of devotion. These messages were not at all unusual and in fact
were very similar to things Mary is reported to have said in other times
and places. They are the kinds of things a priest or pastor says to a con-
gregation, but obviously they carry much greater force if they come from
Mary. People believe that if one listens to Mary's words and follows her
commands, she will act on one's behalf.

What makes Lourdes a successful healing place? I honestly do not
think it is principally because of reports of miraculous physical cures. In
fact, my fellow pilgrims never mentioned them. Most people come to
Lourdes for mental and spiritual renewal, not expecting (although they
may hope for) cures for their physical problems. What I do think is important is that people come expecting healing of some kind, and enough
people find it and pass it on to others in a recurring cycle of bearing witness to what they experienced. Positive feelings are produced and reproduced in a social environment of strong religious faith.

Stories about physical, spiritual, mental, and social healing at Lourdes
accumulate over time and form part of a body of lore. Obviously, only suc-
cesses will be emphasized; one report of a cure is worth many failures or

disappointments (Thomas 1971). And believers do not know or do not care that the facts may become distorted. What happens, over time, is private experiences are transformed by the laity and church authorities into public belief (Zimdars-Swartz 1991). A jumble of stories, true, untrue, or half true, is molded into official versions of events. A mythology emerges that changes ordinary people, places, and events into extraordinary ones that have become "understood truths."

Over a period of five days, I had ample opportunity to observe the behavior of the pilgrims in our group of about forty and to talk to them about their experiences. Our group had various backgrounds (figure 4.1). All, except for myself, were Catholic. A few had simply come out of curiosity, as a side trip on a larger holiday journey through parts of Europe. Several were spending a large part of their annual leave from work. Perhaps a dozen had come one or more times before. One couple had been helpers in the past; this time they were treating themselves and an elderly relative who had been a nun for fifty years to a holiday. One woman, who had been to Lourdes with her former husband, now deceased, came with her teenage son in remembrance. Another woman came to help alleviate the grief she felt over the recent death of her spouse. Some were quite shocked with the rampant commercialism that shattered their preconceived image of this holy place. A few, ironically, were ill much of the week, succumbing in particular to "Lourdes throat," caused probably by pollution from automobiles.

I came to Lourdes as a religious agnostic, not knowing what to expect from what I feared might be a suffocating religious atmosphere. I was relieved to find that my fellow pilgrims did not wear their religion on their sleeves. They did not mind that I was not Catholic. They joked about converting me; however, rather than use aggressive tactics, I think they simply wanted to let Lourdes speak for itself. No one came expecting miracles, although I think most of them believed they could happen. Like many Christians, Protestant or Catholic, they complained about the decaying morals of the modern world. They were basically good people, pillars in small ways within their communities. I felt that they were on a retreat, looking for renewal. Part of the day they were on holiday, having fun, strolling around the shops or having a drink in a bar. At other times they slipped easily into a pious mode and enthusiastically took part in the daily rituals.

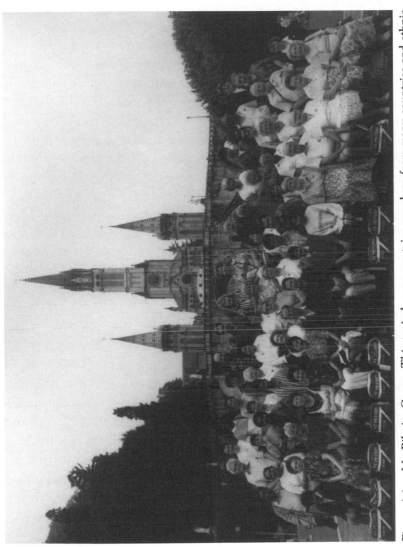

Figure 4.1. My Pilgrim Group. This typical group contains members from many countries and ethnic groups from around the world, drawn together by a common faith and the attraction of a place they have heard about all their lives. Author's photograph.

I can bear witness to the spirit of *communitas* among the group; it was definitely there. People made an effort to include everyone within the group. I submit that it is within a group like ours where a substantial proportion of the real healing that Lourdes is famous for occurs. It was a support group. As the days went by, some members of the group, usually older women, took others under their wing and counseled them. My own favorite "transformation" story is of a young woman who was obviously very distracted and upset when she arrived in Lourdes. She kept to herself at first, but then two or three of the older women began to talk with her. I found out that she lived in a large English city and was overburdened with a stressful family situation. She was totally exhausted from trying to take care of her husband and children. Somehow she got away for a week. As time wore on, she talked more and more with others in the group. It was as though the clouds she came surrounded with had lifted: her physical appearance altered, as did her mental attitude. She had clearly been transformed by the new social relationships she had formed in Lourdes. I have never witnessed such a rapid personality change. My last image of her is chatting gaily with her new friends at the airport as she was about to return to her family.

What Can We Learn from Lourdes?

Once more, at the close of this chapter, I will summarize some of the main ideas that arose from applying four environments to the story of Lourdes. The reader may have noticed that more space was devoted in this chapter to discussions of symbolic and social environments than natural and built environments. The main reason for this is that most people think of the latter environments first when asked about desirable qualities in healing places. I submit that the former environments may be more important in the long run, although they may be more elusive and (say if you are designing a hospital) harder to achieve.

The *natural environment* of Lourdes, set against the background of the Pyrenees, is simply stunning. Apart from the attraction of the grotto to true believers, this is the type of place where many people would go anyway for a holiday. Once again, water plays a major role as it is believed that the springs that Bernadette uncovered with Mary's help have healing power. Like Bath, the town itself spreads out up the steep slopes of hills; like Epidauros, the place is relatively remote from human concentrations. Although the clutter and vulgarity that mark a tourist town detract from the setting, the quiet Domain of Our Lady, with its impressive churches and rapidly flowing river, creates an atmosphere of reverence.

The buildings of Lourdes are not as striking or unique as those found in Epidauros or Bath. I chose rather to focus on a very important aspect of the *built environment* of Lourdes, the contrast between sacred and profane. Even though Lourdes is remote, it juxtaposes vibrant, secular space with awe-inspiring sacred space. My personal experience is that the abrupt transition from one space to the "other" has a profound psychological effect. One can so easily make the journey from the hectic rhythms of daily life to the calming atmosphere of a (w)holy place.

Three aspects of the Lourdes story contribute significantly to its *symbolic environment*. First, there is its pilgrimage origin in the political, religious, and intellectual struggles of the mid-nineteenth century. I would venture to say that Lourdes would not have achieved close to its current reputation if it had not come to symbolize one side in each of these conflicts. Second, beliefs are part of the symbolic environment: at Lourdes it is religious faith that predominates. Millions of believers put credence in miracle cures despite living in an age dominated by biomedicine. Third, the massive pilgrimages to Lourdes create a complex of both concrete (e.g., plastic figurines of Mary) and abstract (e.g., transformation from an old to a new life) symbols in a sacred site.

Lourdes "works" for many people, I believe, because of the *social environment*. Huge crowds are organized in such a way that they engage in a succession of emotionally charged activities. Many achieve a feeling of *communitas* as they travel around with their pilgrim group to sacred spots or mingle with the crowds in daily processions. At Epidauros, Asclepius performed a social function of bridging the gap between the common people and the divine; here Mary and Bernadette together perform a similar task. Lourdes acts as a support system for many who are physically, emotionally, psychologically, or socially ill. Whether they are aware of it or not, the support they are given by those who wish them well may be the chief agent of healing they will experience here.

To conclude the chapter, let us take up briefly the two ideas that were discussed at the end of the preceding chapter, conflict and uniqueness/ generality. Although communitas is what pilgrims strive to achieve at

Lourdes, *conflict* cannot be avoided. Not everyone sees Lourdes (or at least parts of the town) as beautiful, the history of the place is one of struggles among many competing factions, the whole idea of miracle cures is contested, what actually might cure people is debated, and there may be serious rifts among people who work in Lourdes as healers or entrepreneurs. The reputation of the place endures, however, in spite of dissension.

Finally, we take up again the *uniqueness/generality* theme. Every potential healing place achieves success through a unique combination of factors. At Lourdes, religious faith, pilgrimage, stories about successful cures, and daily rituals are some of the components that lead to feelings of well-being. However, although Lourdes's circumstances were very different from those of Bath and Epidauros, it makes similar claims to healing efficacy. The key point is that variations on the same four environments still apply.

CHAPTER FIVE

Therapeutic Hospital Environments

In this chapter we leave historical accounts of healing places behind and concentrate on modern health care facilities. My objective is to show that the healing environments that constituted the framework for the preceding chapters have relevance today. The discussion will usually center on hospitals, although any institution whose purpose is to heal could be considered. In particular, certain long-term care facilities provide good examples of healing environments; they are used here as case studies.

For many, if not most, people a hospital does *not* conjure up images of a healing place, at least not in the broad sense in which we have used the word "healing" in this book. People expect treatment for physical or mental illnesses in hospitals, but rarely anticipate spiritual, emotional, or social healing. In many times and many places hospitals have been looked upon as a last resort or a place where one goes to die. But they are important, they are at the core of our health care system. Can they possibly heal in a holistic way? Fortunately, there are those who think they can. There are many people who work with or in hospitals or live there for a period of time—architects who design buildings, administrators, doctors, nurses, technicians, patients, health policymakers, and academics—who think that hospitals should heal in different ways. What have we learned so far that might help us to think of modern hospitals in terms of healing environments?

In the preceding chapters we looked at three places that achieved a lasting reputation for healing. Little was said about hospitals in these places. Of course, one could think of the Asclepian sanctuary at Epidauros as a kind of specialist clinic where dream healings took place. The novelist Tobias Smollett once called Bath the "great hospital of the nation," and at least one hospital located there contributed to its reputation. Bath General Hospital was founded in 1738 as a hospital for the poor, a move that was intended to control the lower classes, ensure worker productivity, and make the wealthy feel virtuous (Rolls 1998). Evidence from patient records between 1760 and 1789 shows that the hospital was quite successful in treating patients admitted for paralysis from lead poisoning (often caused by drinking cider at harvest time); of the 3,777 cases admitted, 45.4 percent were reported discharged as cured. Bath General became the Royal National Hospital for Rheumatic Diseases in 1935 and achieved notable success in its specialty. Lourdes, too, has its hospitals, but any fame they may have achieved is overshadowed by the pilgrimages to the sacred healing waters in the grotto.

Although hospitals did not figure prominently in discussions of Epidauros, Bath, and Lourdes, there is historical evidence that some people have believed that environments in hospitals should contribute to the therapeutic process. In chapter 1 it was noted that Florence Nightingale (1863) stressed the importance of keeping ward densities low, circulating fresh air, and providing good light and drainage, and promoted several other healthy and hygienic features in hospitals. She argued that the great variations found in hospital mortality rates were due to different built environments. In the eighteenth and nineteenth centuries the idea of *moral treatment* in treating patients as humans as well as treating their diseases led to the establishment of therapeutic communities (Filstead and Rossi 1973). This idea gained its strongest support in places where the mentally ill were treated; three particular places stand out. Geel, Belgium, became a kind of "community hospital" when its residents agreed to take mental patients into their homes. In 1792, at the time of the French Revolution, Philip Pinel created a hospital revolution of his own when he loosed the shackles of inmates in two insane asylums in Paris. In England in 1806, William Tuke established the well-known York Retreat where an atmosphere of kindness and consideration prevailed (Moos 1977).

Attempts continued throughout the nineteenth and twentieth centuries to replace custodial, bureaucratic medical institutions with more open facilities in which patients were encouraged to help themselves throughout the healing process. Perhaps the best example of this idea was the *therapeutic community* or *milieu therapy* movement that began during World War II in Britain (mentioned as an example of social environments in chapter 1) (Filstead and Rossi 1973). Maxwell Jones, who recognized that the problems of many soldiers resulted from environmental stress rather than biological causes, treated 100 soldiers for stress at Maudsley Hospital in London (Jones 1979). In a variety of other hospitals, halfway houses, work places, and even residential communities, the idea of creating groups of patients and caregivers who worked together to heal was put into practice.

Efforts to create therapeutic environments in hospitals appear to come in cycles. In the 1950s, the Nuffield Provincial Hospitals Trust in Britain carried out extensive studies aimed at improving environments in medical institutions (Nuffield 1955). The move to deinstitutionalize the mentally ill that started in the 1960s and 1970s attempted to move people out of large hospitals and into smaller places with more caring environments. At the beginning of the twenty-first century, we are witness to a renewed interest in hospital design (Gesler, Bell, and Curtis 2002). Over the past fifteen years, more than 100 studies carried out in the United States have examined the links between good hospital design and well-being, and in the United Kingdom there is also reemerging interest in creating therapeutic hospital environments (Purvis 2001).

If the ideas about therapeutic environments and healing places that have permeated this book are of any use today, they should apply to modern hospitals. Chapter 1 provided some evidence that they do. In this chapter, I will apply in a systematic way the four healing environments discussed in this book to the study of hospital environments. The goal is to demonstrate that a hospital, that often feared and hated place, *can* achieve a reputation for holistic healing. This will be accomplished by first applying general therapeutic environment ideas to hospitals and then discussing a few detailed case studies.

Bringing Nature to the Hospital

Many people involved in trying to make hospitals a healing place retain the age-old belief that nature heals. This belief can be seen most simply in the daily ritual of bringing flowers to a recovering patient. At times, nature is very consciously brought within a hospital's walls (Gerlach-Spriggs, Kaufman, and Warner 1998). A cancer treatment center, for example, has a garden atrium planted with seasonal flowers and plants (Scott 1992). The operating theaters at the Woodwinds Hospital in Minneapolis are furnished with backlit photographs of woodlands and rushing waters (Purvis 2001). Hospitals may also be situated within nature, so that patients look out onto or are surrounded by elements of the natural environment. In chapter 1, the example was given of research that showed that patients who looked out on trees as opposed to a brick wall had a faster and more pleasant recovery from gall bladder surgery (Ulrich 1984). Kearns (1991) writes of the therapeutic effect on Maori patients of a magnificent view from a hospital in Hokianga, New Zealand. Every patient at the Baptist Health Medical Center in North Little Rock, Arkansas, has a porch with a view of a forest.

The point was made in preceding chapters that remoteness was often an asset to the healing process. As an example, situating mental health hospitals in rural areas was extolled by planners involved in the "mad-business" of the nineteenth century (Philo 1987). The belief was that people with mental illness could not cope with the urban environments of the new industrial society and would only recover in peaceful, natural surroundings. Of course, hospitals built in remote places are not readily accessible to rapidly growing urban populations throughout the world today. One can achieve a kind of remoteness in an urban setting by ensuring privacy for patients, but this is an expensive proposition and unreasonable in most situations. The solution in most cases is to bring nature to the hospital and attempt to create a feeling of getting away from it all that a natural setting engenders.

Building Design as Therapy

I venture to say that most people, when asked what features of a hospital might be therapeutic, would mention elements of the built environment. One could, of course, include such "natural" features as a garden atrium as part of this environment. As mentioned in chapter 1, most people respond favorably or unfavorably to things they can see, hear, smell, taste, or touch (Hutton and Richardson 1995). These are the kinds of features that have interested environmental psychologists, the primary investigators of built environments, over several decades (Holahan 1979; Reizenstein 1982; Spencer and Blades 1986).

A wide range of specific features of the built hospital environment could be studied: cleanliness, spaciousness, lighting, color, ventilation, temperature, and the effects of weather, to name a few (Macdonald et al. 1981; Williams 1988). Several studies have demonstrated that noise levels (e.g., from equipment or staff conversations) can be of sufficient intensity to interfere with patients' sleep and rest (Griffin 1992). The *lack* of sensory stimuli may also have a deleterious effect on health. Wilson (1972), comparing postoperative surgical patients in two hospitals, found that the group that had no windows in their rooms had higher rates (40 percent) of postoperative delirium than a matched group who had windows (18 percent).

In contrast to social and symbolic environments, natural and built environments in hospitals can be studied more easily using quantifiable data. There is a rather extensive literature that attempts to analyze the effects of specific design features on patient and staff behavior. To take just one example, a study compared three nursing units in a hospital: two were not altered; the third was renovated (Becker 1977). Results of a before and after survey showed that changes in the renovated unit had a positive effect on the mood and morale of staff. In this unit, there were also significant changes in the movement of patients and staff: more people went to places where they could interact with others more easily and the overall level of activity was increased.

Some aspects of the built environment are not as easily measured. Yi-Fu Tuan (1974) speaks of the meaning that "public symbols" such as the Vietnam War Memorial in Washington, D.C., or the site of the former World Trade Center in Manhattan have for people. Public symbols may inspire feelings of identity, solidarity, or comfort. For some, hospital buildings, if their architecture is impressive, may engender these kinds of feelings. Indeed, places such as Rochester, Minnesota (home of the Mayo Clinic), have come to be identified by their hospitals.

The field of proxemics is especially pertinent to the geographical study of built environments in hospitals as it looks at the spatial aspects of human behavior (Stokols 1978). Studies guided by proxemics have examined the effects of *density* or people per unit of space as well as *crowding* or the psychological effects of perceiving that there are too many people in a space. Other studies have focused on the concept of territoriality and asked how people stake out personal spaces or react to a lack of privacy (Russel and Ward 1982; Williams 1988). Becker (1977) and Holahan (1979) both made maps of where groups of patients were at different times; the maps provided valuable information on where patients tended to spend time and interact with others. A study carried out almost four decades ago (Rosengren and DeVault 1963) also looked at patient movements. Following the travels of women in an obstetrical hospital, the researchers showed that patients behaved very differently in different rooms as well as at different stages in the birthing process.

Interpreting Symbols in Hospitals

The things people experience with their senses in a hospital (or anywhere) create meanings for them beyond surface appearances (Canter and Canter 1979). Furthermore, what people see, hear, touch, taste, or smell in a hospital produces different meanings, depending on their cultural heritage and past experiences. Human activity is often based on images rather than objective reality, an idea that advertisers capitalize on. Put another way, symbols mediate between a stimulus and a response (Evans 1982). To cite a well-known example, a patient sees a doctor's white coat (which might symbolize purity, honesty, or competence) and responds with respect and compliance.

In this section I highlight those ideas and objects that often lie hidden and whose effects are difficult to measure, but are nonetheless potentially very important in affecting human attitudes and behavior in hospital settings. The most easily noticed symbols in a hospital are physical objects. I have already discussed the positive human response to such natural features as water and trees and to the feelings of security and identity that an imposing hospital building might engender. The high-tech equipment that hospitals see as essential to remain competitive can evince extreme feelings; people are frightened or impressed by equipment that ranges from a syringe to an MRI scanner (Kenny and Canter 1979). The signs along hospital corridors that direct patients and staff to various medical departments are often a very significant aspect of the symbolic environment. Most of us have probably found hospital signage very bewildering; imagine what someone who cannot even read the signs must feel.

Ideas that circulate within hospitals are harder to grasp than physical objects, but their effect may be extremely important. One prominent type of idea is the beliefs various people have about health issues such as what causes a certain illness and what is the best way to treat it. These beliefs are called *explanatory models* (Good 1994; Kleinman 1978) and have been used extensively by medical anthropologists to help explain the behavior of medical personnel and patients. If a patient and his/her doctor have similar explanatory models, this may aid the healing process. Unfortunately, the models of laypeople and medical experts often clash and thereby inhibit healing. Within hospital settings, the explanatory model notion has been studied rather extensively by researchers who have very carefully examined doctor-patient consultations. Studies have shown that doctors often dominate these conversations, but also how some patients resist domination and attempt to make their true feelings known (Mishler 1984; Todd and Fisher 1993).

There are many other ideas besides explanatory models that play important roles in hospital settings. For example, people have certain expectations about the care they will receive when they come to a hospital; these may either be confirmed or unfulfilled (Hutton and Richardson 1995). Those who placed valuable artworks in the Chelsea and Westminster Hospital in London obviously had the idea that art was therapeutic. Not everyone will like a particular piece of work, however. As an example, Chelsea and Westminster was given an artwork by the controversial artist Damien Hirst that features a human figure with a staring single eye and exposed internal organs (Gibbons 2001). Cornish (1997) reports that an asylum that closed down evoked two contrasting responses: many former patients had very positive feelings about the place because it symbolized refuge and security, whereas outsiders stigmatized it because it represented a feared "other." Becker (1977) discovered that people reacted favorably to design changes in a hospital because they thought the changes made it look more "modern." In their examination of the Starship Hospital for children in Auckland, Kearns and Barnett (1999) showed that the spaceship concept signified adventure to the patients and helped them to overcome their fears. "Starship" is also symbolic of Enterprise, with reference both to the Star Trek television series and a commercial venture.

All the examples cited in the preceding paragraph illustrate how "stories" are told about hospitals, whether by patients commenting on their experiences or by hospital staff and promoters who wish to enhance the reputation of their institution. Some of these stories may even achieve the status of myth. Take, for example, the reputation of the Mayo Clinic in Rochester, Minnesota. The father of a colleague is probably quite typical in his feelings about the place. He tried unsuccessfully for many years to cure his chronic illness, making the rounds of several physicians prominent in their field, and then went to the Mayo Clinic and was healed. He now speaks of the place with reverence and awe. I do not dispute that the clinic's reputation is well deserved; nonetheless, Mayo has perpetuated a story about itself that is somehow larger than life.

Gifford and Mullner write:

> The institutional nature of hospitals allows them to build community alliances and recreate myths of meaning for internal and external public legitimization. In this sense, hospitals can manipulate culture by producing images of themselves aimed at gaining community support. (1988, 1290)

As an example of this idea, hospitals at the beginning of the twentieth century successfully projected an image of hope to the desperately ill. A more specific example of hospital entrepreneurship is Duke Medical School in Durham, North Carolina. This hospital complex attracts leading specialists from all over the world and has achieved a widespread reputation for specialist care, enhanced by self-promotion. Durham itself has been promoted as the "City of Medicine." Durham is certainly not the "City of Health," as one can easily perceive on visits to the shabbier parts of town where low-income African Americans, recently arrived Hispanics, and European Americans reside.

Rituals are another important component of symbolic environments. Simple hospital-based examples would be bringing flowers or gifts to a patient or the comforting words of a religious counselor. When doctors make case presentations on their rounds they use a standard format and stylized vocabulary. Certain words are used repeatedly and the patient being discussed is labeled in typical ways. Case presentations allow senior physicians to display their knowledge and are also used to socialize interns into new ways of speaking and thinking (Anspach 1988). Rituals are also essential in dictating operating room etiquette (Katz 1981). On the surface, the elaborate cleansing techniques that surgeons and their assistants use are to prevent infections, but they also help medical personnel to cope with uncertain situations. Words such as "clean" or "contaminated" take on different meanings at different stages during an operation. There are appropriate times and places for complete silence, small talk, or jokes.

Fostering Social Relationships

Hospitals are gathering places for a wide variety of people who play many different roles. In such situations, how well people get along with each other is important, especially to the health of patients, but also to everyone else's health and well-being. Unfortunately, social relationships are often not at their best in hospitals. As we noted above, doctors may dominate patients and suppress their attempts to express themselves. Hospitals are also well known for fostering status hierarchies of personnel, from the cleaning staff on up to surgeons and administrators. The leaders of the therapeutic community movement mentioned in the introduction to this chapter recognized that social structures were important to health. To combat inequalities, four basic themes were developed: (1) democratization, (2) permissiveness, (3) reality confrontation, and (4) communalism (Morrice 1979). These themes were fostered by such practices as facilitating communication, breaking down hierarchies of authority, staff/patient consensus in decision making, and providing living-learning experiences.

How does one go about assessing the social environment of a hospital? Moos (1977) attempted to do this using the concept of a *social climate* that he categorized into four factors. First is the institutional context that includes such items as the type of ownership (e.g., public or private), size, and staffing (e.g., mix of generalists and specialists). Second are physical and architectural features, what we have been calling the built environment (and which we certainly acknowledge affects the social environment). Third is hospital organization, including such things as choices available to patients and the degree to which they participate in the healing process. Fourth are group characteristics: age, gender, ethnicity, and level of impairment, as examples. This way of setting out the parameters of a social climate lends itself to measurement. Thus Flarey (1991) used the ideas developed by Moos and colleagues to construct a work environment scale that was used in nursing administration research.

We all like to "be in control of the situation" and this is never truer than in a hospital setting. Individual control of course has to be seen in relation to others, so it is also a social phenomenon. The degree of autonomy or control that staff and patients can experience has been studied fairly extensively. Noise of any type can inhibit healing, but Minckley (1968) confirmed what many of us feel: noise is especially disturbing to patients if they cannot identify the source. Introducing new technologies may have the effect of reducing patient control (Kenny and Canter 1979): think of the classic image portrayed in the television drama *ER* of a patient totally captured in a web of tubes and monitors, a hybrid human/machine. When Ryden (1985) examined support for autonomy among older adults in four proprietary nursing homes, she discovered that caregivers often expressed their need for control, but seldom emphasized choices for their patients. Patients who experienced a lack of control over their daily activities became demoralized and felt powerless.

Social environments in hospitals have been studied in a number of interesting ways. Leatt and Schneck (1982) examined similarities and differences in the work environments of nine types of nursing subunits, using measures of autonomy, complexity, and interactions with people outside the subunits. Different nursing styles in maternity wards have been found to affect the way women interact with their newborn babies (Porter and Watson 1985). Holahan (1979) compared patient behavior in an old ward and a remodeled one and found that the latter stimulated more social interactions among patients and staff. All these studies indicate that social environments in hospitals can be changed to influence the healing process.

Case Studies

Each of the preceding sections dealt with one of the four healing environments that form the core of this book. Here, I look at one hospital and two long-term care facilities that illustrate how all four environments can be examined within one place. These case studies indicate that the concepts developed throughout the book can truly be realized and integrated within a modern health care setting.

Glasgow Homoeopathic Hospital

The planners of the Glasgow Homoeopathic Hospital (GHH) in Scotland consciously tried to create a place with environments conducive to healing (Macmon 2001). This facility is a small, fifteen-bed hospital that provides outpatient consulting and physiotherapy; later it will include academic facilities as well. Interestingly, the project was the result of an Open Design Competition that was won in 1995 by the architectural firm Maclachlan Monaghan, which changed its name in July 2001 to Macmon chartered architects. The designers worked closely with patient user groups and clinicians with the intent to create a holistic environment. Their goal was to provide "The very highest commitment to the creation of a place of healing and beauty, commensurate with Homoeopathic, care philosophies" within strict cost limits (Macmon 2001, 2) (figure 5.1).

The natural environment of GHH consists of a therapy garden surrounded by a courtyard, a water therapy facility, and outdoor landscaping. Typically, a great deal of attention was paid to the built environment. The design attempted to maximize natural lighting and ventilation. Full-spectrum, high-frequency fluorescent lights, adapted to shield people from electromagnetic emissions, were installed. To cut costs, the geometry of the first phase of building was rectilinear, but curvilinear "organic" features were used in strategic areas, and subsequent design elements will be more free-form. Like the Greek builders at Epidauros, the architects attempted to integrate buildings and landscape.

At least two aspects of GHH form part of a symbolic environment. One is the homoeopathic beliefs held by clinicians and patients that often run counter to biomedicine and are espoused as holistic, providing different dimensions of healing for the whole person. Also, an artist, Jane Kelly, was invited to collaborate over color strategies and furniture selection. In addition, she developed and then implemented the therapy garden. The creation of a social environment is especially interesting. Since the site is bounded by "imposing, if not hostile" features (a railway track, an estate boiler house, a public footpath, and town housing), ancillary accommodation is located along the boundary as a physical and visual defense. At the same time, glazed screens that open along the inner perimeter wall provide a link to the landscape and thus mitigate potential feelings of isolation. In other words, attention to inside and outside spaces and the links between them provides a sense of a community protected from outside disturbances and at the same time a feeling of access to the world outside the hospital (Macmon 2001).

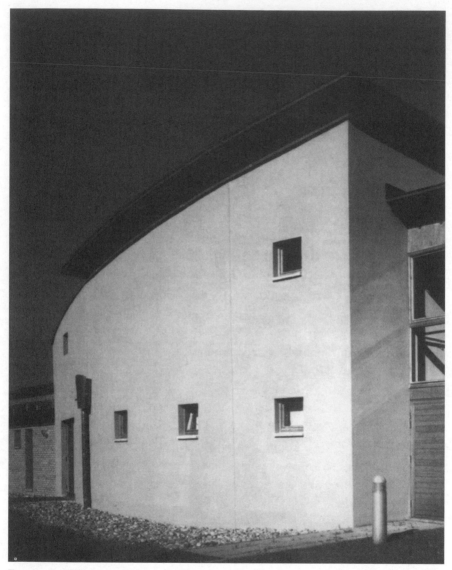

Figure 5.1. Glasgow Homoeopathic Hospital. Designed by Maclachlan Monaghan, architects. Courtesy of Macmon chartered architects, Glasgow, Scotland.

Designing to Accommodate Persons with Alzheimer's

There are around 1.6 million Americans in nursing homes; about half of them suffer from Alzheimer's disease or other forms of dementia. Taking care of people with Alzheimer's is particularly difficult as they have a decreased attention span and tend to wander because they have lost the ability to absorb the meaning of images and words. The frustrating paradox is that they seek stimulus but cannot handle too much of it. They appear to be relentlessly searching for "home," a place of security, familiarity, and identity. Nursing homes, unfortunately, are usually not designed to cope with this problem. Some institutions have restrained Alzheimer's residents or used "chemical constraints." Most homes simply are not designed to handle the bewilderment and paranoia that Alzheimer's engenders (Gladwell 1997).

Presbyterian SeniorCare, a nonprofit long-term care group in western Pennsylvania, opened Woodside Place in the Pittsburgh suburb of Oakmont to deal with the seemingly insurmountable problems Alzheimer's causes. Their goal was to "create a space that allowed for movement with meaning, that allowed patients to explore and then—just as important— allowed them to find their way home again" (Gladwell 1997, 137). In the words of a staff member: "[p]laces like Woodside are creatively and innovatively dealing with the huge challenges of the disease. It's really all about thinking out of the box, getting away from the medical model and letting people live freely within the walls of Woodside Place" (personal communication with Anna Scott of SeniorCare 2002).

Woodside Place is situated on a small wooded lot behind a larger nursing home. Big picture windows allow for easy viewing access to the outdoors. Care is taken, however, not to make nature too overwhelming. If trees or shrubs grow too big, they can create too much stimulus, so they are cut back. A plant that looks like a person can cause anxiety and must be reshaped. In other words, a natural environment is present, but it is altered to accommodate a particular form of cognitive impairment caused by brain disease.

The Oakmont facility is designed to resemble a traditional Pennsylvania Shaker Village (figure 5.2). Three high-roofed, gray-shingled houses accommodate three groups of twelve residents each. Keeping the number of patients low is comforting and nonthreatening. The buildings are mostly carpeted. The walls are painted in neutral colors; many have

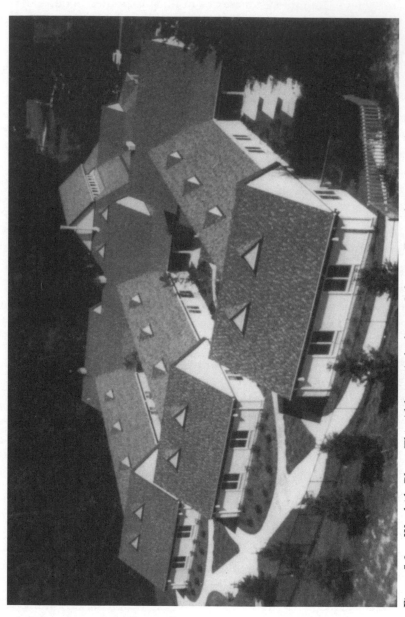

Figure 5.2. Woodside Place. This Alzheimer's facility in Oakmont, Pennsylvania, is run by Presbyterian Senior-Care. The cluster of buildings is modeled after a Pennsylvania Shaker Village. The design produces a comfortable and intimate environment for residents. Courtesy of Presbyterian SeniorCare, Oakmont, Pennsylvania.

textured wallpaper to elicit tactile responses. Staff do not work in an office or from a nursing station, but in the kitchen, which becomes both hearth and home. Cooking smells permeate the house: this is important because the sense of smell is one of the last faculties to leave a person with Alzheimer's.

Images encountered in the typical hospital are especially frightening to people with Alzheimer's. A physician's white coat may remind one of medical crises suffered in the past; a nurse's voice over the intercom may signify a terrifying, disembodied presence; a long, straight corridor may present an impossible challenge. Taking these problems with the symbolic environment into account, SeniorCare tried to deinstitutionalize Woodside Place. Attention was given to design features that might cause concern. For example, because the windows created potentially threatening shadows in the evening (someone out to get a patient, perhaps), recessed lighting was installed to eliminate most of the shadows. Some features are intended to provide subtle symbolic stimuli. The hallways leading from the houses to the main building (which has a music room, a television room, and a meeting hall) are tiled to create a contrast to the carpeted houses, signal arrival in a public space, and provide tactile and acoustical differentiation. The floors are a combination of tile, carpeting, and vinyl that looks like hardwood floors. The heating system is in the floors so that people can go barefoot if they like and pick up clues as to where they are (Scott 2002).

Patients with Alzheimer's lose their identity and become very individualistic in their behavior. Many are asleep or awake or eat at odd hours. Creating social cohesion among residents is therefore a serious challenge. Woodside Place meets the challenge in innovative ways. Residents are not regimented, they are free to move around in familiar environments. Resident numbers are not overwhelming. Meals are served around the clock; residents who forgot they had breakfast already may have the meal five or six times before lunch. As mentioned above, life centers around the kitchen. Evidently, efforts to create a homelike environment have been successful, as an independent study carried out by the graduate schools of the University of Pittsburgh and Carnegie Mellon shows that residents spend three times as much time socializing with other residents in a homelike atmosphere than those in a traditional nursing home (Gladwell 1997). In addition, they progress more slowly in their disease, stay physically active longer, and their care costs are lower than their counterparts' (McGrath 2002).

The Green House Project for Long-Term Care

It is often said that long-term care in the United States and other countries is in desperate need of reform. The designers of the Green House Project (GHP) have declared that: "The time has come to reinvent the long-term care environment for the 21st century. We must change the way we think about, regulate and deliver services to people who are frail, disabled or elderly" (GHP 2002, 1). The project is currently attempting to "design, build and test a radically new approach to residential long-term care for the elderly" (2). How does it propose to do this in light of our four environments?

GHP is planning a built environment that resembles that of Woodside Place, discussed in the preceding case study. Forty-two elderly and disabled people from Utica, New York, will be moved out of a nursing facility and into seven Green Houses. The houses are designed to fit into neighborhoods so well that someone driving along the street could not tell which ones were Green. The intention is to create a feeling of warmth within each house through the floor plan, furnishings, décor, and a careful choice of staff. Technology will be introduced that is unobtrusive and yet "ensures safety, promotes quality of care, rigor in record keeping, and community and family involvement" (GHP 2002, 2).

The natural environment that GHP envisions is based on the simple statement that the Green Houses older persons live in must be green. The designers believe that humans need close and continuing contact with the living world. They recognize that quality of life is promoted by providing older persons with an environment that includes green plants, animals, and the laughter of children.

GHP is a reaction against the cold, sterile, bureaucratic environments that too often prevail in long-term care institutions. Personnel are attempting to create social environments that maintain the freedom and independence of individuals as much as possible. Cold is to be replaced by warmth through building design and an emphasis on tolerance, patience, forgiveness, and respect for human relationships. Like the therapeutic community movement mentioned earlier in this chapter, GHP strives to break down the hierarchical "chains of command" that staff in many institutions are socialized into following. Specialists trained in quality long-term care will enter Green Houses as experts and advisors, not bosses. The rules and regulations that provide a refuge from the difficulty of establishing and maintaining social relationships in many places will be replaced by informality and personal commitments to the elderly and their needs. The problem of social isolation will be tackled with an outreach program to the surrounding neighborhood.

The concepts of greenness and warmth already discussed are an essential part of GHP's symbolic environment. Plants, animals, and children are symbols of life that counteract the atmosphere of disease and death that can so easily permeate a long-term care facility. The warmth created by caring staff gives meaning to the lives of older persons. What I find of particular symbolic importance is the use (or disuse) of recent technologies. The use of videotaped surveillance is forbidden because it erodes trust (and can lead to problems with legal liability). In contrast, a Web cam approach is being used whereby family members, health professionals, and others can "stop by" via Internet and visit residents any time, day or night. This, of course, should not replace the vitally important personal visit.

Conclusion

Hospitals, as well as other health care facilities, have a serious image problem. Although they are places where physical healing takes place, often with the help of seemingly miraculous modern technology and expertise, they rarely have a reputation for healing mentally, spiritually, or socially. It is to be hoped that this chapter has shown that hospitals *can* become places that heal in different ways. For this to happen, I argue, attention has to shift from currently dominant concerns such as cost-cutting (which often is counterproductive in the long run), high-tech equipment (which is expensive and diverts resources away from more important needs), and a focus on physical healing only (which neglects other types of healing) to more holistic attitudes toward the healing process. Furthermore, improvements in hospital environments must not only be made to make patients "feel better," although that is very important. To be truly effective, changes must alter hospital "cultures." If the prevailing culture within a hospital is focused mainly on physical healing, cost-cutting efficiency, and a blind worship of the gods of technology, I believe that culture should be changed.

Although modern hospitals may seem a far cry from the Asclepian sanctuary at Epidauros, the mineral springs at Bath, or the grotto at Lourdes, one can discuss them in terms of the same kinds of healing environments or at least the potential for them. Ideas about these environments are not new. Periodically, it seems, a few individuals attempt to reform the atmosphere of hospitals and other institutions that provide healing by looking beyond strictly biomedical, technological, or economic concerns.

Looking at hospitals through the lenses of our four environments permits us to make some practical suggestions for enhancing the healing potential of hospitals. Nature can be brought into hospitals through the introduction of plants (and perhaps animals such as dogs and cats), water displays, or pictures of outdoor scenes. In addition, hospitals can be surrounded by nature through careful landscape design. There are many specific items of the built environment that can aid the healing process, including both imposing and pleasing facades, letting in lots of light and air, controlling noise and smells, and providing wall colors and works of art that are soothing to the eye and mind. I would argue that perhaps most attention should be paid to symbolic environments because they are usually neglected. The suggestion here is that hospital staff try to understand what various aspects of the hospital setting—building design, beliefs about disease, feelings about various pieces of equipment, the language used in consultations—mean to people because these meanings affect their thinking and behavior. Finally, social environments can be improved by paying more attention to communications between all the actors on the hospital stage, fostering patient participation, and breaking down status hierarchies.

The case studies discussed above demonstrate that specific features of the four environments have consciously been used by health facility planners to aid in the healing process. This is certainly encouraging. A question that many readers might ask, however, is whether or not these features could easily be implemented in other healing places. After all, the examples are based on unusually dedicated and highly motivated practitioners taking care of small groups of people. It would be almost impossible to transfer the feelings of warmth that these places provide to large hospital wards. In addition, facilities such as Woodside Place or the

Green Houses are costly. A start has to be made, however. Large hospital units can be split up into more "cozy" segments. If the societal will is there, funds can be diverted from costly programs such as national defense or building prisons to provide quality health care for all. Furthermore, many of the features discussed in the case studies (e.g., landscaping, breaking down status hierarchies, Web visits), although they may be difficult to implement, could be tried. In short, we know what to do and it has been done in certain places; now the lessons learned have to be expanded throughout the health care system.

Let me end this chapter by raising three issues that four colleagues and I are beginning to address. We recognize that, increasingly, hospitals and other health facilities are incorporating what they believe to be healing design features. It is appropriate, therefore, to critically review these features. First we must examine the sources of information that architects and others use to design hospitals or other care facilities. Where do their ideas come from? Do they focus on costs, efficiency, holistic concepts, the natural sciences, the social sciences, or the humanities? Second we must discern who participates in molding hospital environments. When plans are made to design or redesign a hospital or a hospital wing, which groups of people are involved: architects, administrators, staff, or patients? One suspects that patients and many staff members have little say in the matter and yet they are the very people the hospital should be serving. Third we must look at the equity in the evaluation of hospital design features. Within the overall hospital culture there are many subcultures. We have to be very sensitive to how people of different ethnicity, gender, ability, age, and religion interpret and experience the four hospital environments. This means asking them for their reactions to such things as signage or works of art, certainly not an easy task, but one that should be carried out.

CHAPTER SIX

☙

Conclusion

In this concluding chapter, rather than providing another set of summary statements to add to those set out at the ends of the preceding chapters, I decided to write a few short essays or reflections on what I have learned in working with healing places. Each essay stands on its own, but some threads of meaning flow from one to the next.

Feeling Better and Changing Cultures

What is the purpose of introducing a specific aspect of a therapeutic environment to a place in which healing is supposed to be taking place? A simple answer is that we want to make patients "feel better" (Miles 1997). This is certainly a worthy goal and it resonates with the claim that enhancing emotional and mental states can aid in physical healing.

Certainly we want patients to feel better and it seems churlish to question this goal. However, a little thought leads one to think of other goals that might be masked by this one. Keeping patients feeling good might be part of an attempt to control them, to keep them docile, to prevent them from raising questions about their diagnoses or treatments. Of course, keeping patients under control could contribute to improving the health of staff, certainly a desirable goal for the latter.

This discussion about making patients feel better leads us to ask what other goals people might have in mind for features that are represented as being therapeutic. One goal could be efficiency; a change in ward design, for example, could enable nurses to reach patients more quickly and that could have a healing effect. Efficiency, however, can produce results that are counter to healing. A famous example is waking up patients to give them medications; this fits into the nursing schedule, but it severely disturbs the patients' needed rest.

A very good reason for landscaping a healing institution or building an inspiring facade could be to promote the place. Singh (1990) notes that there is a growing trend toward "marketization" of the health care industry and suggests that patients will be attracted to a hospital if they are satisfied with different "objects" (e.g., doctors and nurses) as well as such things as access and costs. More specifically, Kearns and Barnett (1999) show how a spaceship motif was used by a hospital in Auckland to sell the place to children and their parents. One could say, of course, that marketing healing places brings in needed funds for therapeutic purposes and thereby contributes to health. Selling places, however, can also detract from patient care. Designs that catch the eye and open pocketbooks may paper over, for example, negative physician attitudes toward patients.

What I am implying in this discussion of goals is that, although making patients happy, achieving efficiency, or marketing can have healing effects, the most important goal to my way of thinking lies in a different direction. In a perceptive chapter on the use of art works in the health services, Malcolm Miles suggests that a worthy goal might be a change in health care culture. He writes: "[Art] may be either a cultural addition to hospital environments, or part of a change in the culture of health care" (1997, 150).

So the big question for me is, how can specific elements of healing environments be brought to bear on changing institutional cultures? What is the point of buying an expensive painting for display in a hospital lobby if many people dislike it, find no meaning in it, or actually become ill thinking about it? One solution to this problem is to have patients and staff (as opposed to management, an art committee, or donors seeking publicity) help select the art. Other suggestions are made in the "How to Do It" section below.

The Two Cultures

There are two places I go for health care on a regular basis: once a year to a physician in a group practice for a check-up and several times a year to a chiropractor for treatment and maintenance for a chronic lower back problem. The doctor's office is in a fairly new building set in a grove of trees in a quiet part of town, some distance down the road from a large teaching hospital complex. The reception areas and waiting room are spacious and comfortable, but devoid of much stimulus other than medical and news magazines. The nurses are efficient but not especially friendly and waiting times are tolerable. I found, after some searching, a doctor within the practice that seems genuinely interested in my welfare, although I spend only about ten minutes a year with him. What is really unpleasant about this practice is the handling of patients and their paperwork at the admissions and exit desks. Simply put, the workers there are almost invariably rude; they often make my blood boil. Tension is often in the air around these desks as patients and staff often misunderstand each other and quarrel. This is not a therapeutic environment and it affects one's entire experience of the place.

In contrast, I look forward to going to the chiropractor. He shares an establishment with several small rooms with a fellow D.C. in a medium-sized shopping mall at the edge of a woods. There is a fish tank in the waiting room and also books and crayons for children who come with their patient parents or to be treated themselves. There is a fairly wide range of magazines to browse, including some on preventive care. The treatment room is "open"; that is, one can see others being manipulated and talk to still others while waiting for treatment. Most important is the social environment: the staff is just as busy as they are at the physician group practice, but they are invariably helpful and friendly. A patient can relax in this atmosphere. I was wary of the open treatment plan at first, but came to appreciate the social interaction.

What makes these two healing places different? It is not that one office is nonbiomedical and the other biomedical because I have been in D.C.'s offices where the atmosphere was cold and tense and there are aspects of my interactions with M.D.s in their offices that have been very positive. The difference, I feel, hinges upon local cultures. The biomedical group practice is favored in its natural and built environments (with the exception of the aquarium), and both have good potential for social and symbolic environments to aid in healing. But workers in the chiropractic office put their environments to better use. The D.C. talks to children about the fish; patients and staff move about freely and discuss their ailments as well as other aspects of their daily lives. Watching someone else get adjusted on what at first glance may be a forbidding "workbench" makes a patient more comfortable with the technique. To summarize, one culture invokes tension, the other relaxation.

In his book, *The Tipping Point*, Malcolm Gladwell (2000) suggests that little things can make a big difference in promoting a new idea. I think this concept could be put to good use in changing institutional health cultures. A little thing like a fish tank can really change an atmosphere. Kearns and Barnett (1997) report that patients in low-cost clinics in New Zealand say that waiting room ambience (e.g., magazines, television, smells) is more important than cost. Among several specialist clinics at our local hospital, one stands out as having an atmosphere of conviviality. I trace the cheery greetings by the receptionists, the caring attitude of the nurses, and the continual chatter and laughter among the staff to one or two of the physicians who project an aura of good feeling. Once the will is there, one strong push can tip the balance from a nontherapeutic to a therapeutic environment.

The Four Environments

Something that I had hoped for, but not really expected, was that there would be a few types of environments that played significant roles in all of the three healing places as well as in hospitals. As I worked through the material, I kept changing what seemed to be the common environments (perhaps seven or eight in total were considered) until the ones discussed throughout the book made it to the final four. Now I would like to ask two further questions about the four environments. Which are the most important? Which are the easiest to achieve?

Let us start with the latter question first. I would guess that most people who think about designing or evaluating a healing place would think first about natural and built environments. Landscaping, bringing nature into the hospital, imposing facades: these are the kinds of things that get talked about. Natural and built environments are often visual, although the other senses might also be involved. They catch the eye, they are relatively easy to sell to the public and prospective donors. Because of their visibility and because their healing potential is relatively easy for many people to understand (e.g., nature heals, air and light are good for both body and soul), building elements and objects from nature would seem the easiest to incorporate into designs.

But are natural and built environments as important as social and symbolic ones? This of course is a loaded question. "Important in what way?" one might ask. What is important for me is the overall healing process, which includes physical, mental, spiritual, and emotional healing. For that, I suggest that symbolic and social environments are more important. This is a hard statement to prove. Social and symbolic environments are more abstract; they tend to engage the mind rather than the senses. Their effects are harder to measure and they are definitely harder to achieve. And yet I hope that this book has gone some way in convincing the reader of their importance. Furthermore, if they are the more important environments, designers of healing places need to pay more attention to them.

The distinction between natural and built environments versus social and symbolic environments is similar to the distinction between feeling better and changing cultures. Changes in the former two environments are more likely to make people feel better, although they could also help to change institutional culture. In contrast, to really change cultures I believe one has to alter social and symbolic environments. Changing staff morale is more likely to be achieved through lessening status hierarchies than placing a fountain in the foyer. Understanding and sympathizing with a patient's explanatory model is more helpful to a patient than an imposing hospital facade.

The built/natural versus symbolic/social distinction can also be examined through the lens of Tuan's (1974) discussion of *public symbols* versus *fields of care*. The former appeals mainly to our visual sense and has a direct and immediate effect. Public symbols often inspire awe and include such things as statues of war heroes and massive buildings. In contrast, fields of care tend to be taken in by the nonvisual senses: hearing, touch, taste, and smell. They can only be known through long experience and tend to inspire affection rather than awe. They often involve networks of interpersonal concern such as those found in a close-knit neighborhood or an intensive care unit in a hospital. There is some correspondence, I think, between natural and built environments and public symbols and between symbolic and social environments and fields of care. I would also relate public symbols to making patients feel better and fields of care to changing healing cultures.

Pilgrimages, Myths, and Everyday Rituals

The point has been made that it is not so much the specifics of the four environments applied to healing places that is important but rather the framework and concepts they offer. Still, there are a few especially intriguing ideas that arose in the course of my study of Epidauros, Bath, Lourdes, and hospitals that could be applied to potentially healing places in imaginative ways. Here are three suggestions.

A physician who heard me lecture on therapeutic landscapes made the observation that many patients that he consults appear to be on a pilgrimage. This does not mean that they have come to him seeking miracle cures like many who travel to Lourdes. He contends, however, that they are on a quest. They left their homes and made a journey, usually not over a long distance, to confront an illness with a physician's help. Their goal was to somehow transform their illness into a cure or at least into something manageable. What a valuable insight into the healing process: healing as the outcome of a pilgrimage that intimately involves patient and practitioner.

I find it remarkable that Epidauros, Bath, and Lourdes all had myths that added to their reputations for healing. Stories about Asclepius's parentage, King Bladud's leprosy cure, and Bernadette's saintly life are important aspects of the symbolic landscapes of those places. Myths can reveal hidden meanings that do not appear on the surface. They symbolize what people feel is really important in their relationship to the physical environment, their interactions with other people, and with the supernatural. They are stories told about the world that become understood truths.

Are there modern myths about health? I think so. It is hard to think of detailed stories such as those connected with the three historic healing places. However, I believe that when medical science promotes itself by telling stories of, say, miraculous cancer cures, it is helping to create a myth that it has all the answers. If one did a survey that asked people why tuberculosis declined so dramatically during the twentieth century, many people would probably say it was because of antibiotics. However, the evidence suggests that the decline began before antibiotics were introduced and was due to higher standards of living that included improved measures of public health. The tuberculosis myth should focus on Asclepius's daughter Hygieia rather than on Asclepius.

There are many other myths besides biomedical ones. Promoters of alternative or complementary health care tell stories about the miraculous healing powers of certain herbs or practices that remind one of the snake oil salesmen who traveled throughout the United States in the nineteenth century. Both positive and negative myths grow up around the care one receives in a hospital, based on one or two incidents that spread quickly through the rumor mill.

Whether they are used consciously or not, myths have the power to form or change perceptions. It is essential to look for the stories that say so much about what people feel is important (or are persuaded to feel is important) in health care. When myths are false or hide the truth, this should be pointed out. Perhaps we can even tell stories that point toward new truths: stories about prevention being more important than cure, stories about how the mind and the body work together, stories about efficacious complementary medicines, stories about successful healing places.

Hospitals can be frightening places because patients are forced to live in environments that are unfamiliar and over which they have little control. At home, we are comforted by daily routines and rituals. The hospital has its rituals, too, but they are usually not ours. One of the lessons learned from studying healing places is that incorporating the familiar as well as daily routines can aid the healing process. At Epidauros, people carried out many of the same activities they pursued at home, albeit in an atmosphere heightened by the sacred and mysterious. Social activities at Bath were deliberately routinized. My experience at Lourdes told me that fellow pilgrims were comforted by such daily activities as eating, talking, and going to Mass.

We can of course bring the familiar into the hospital in the form of pictures of loved ones or bits of reading material. Hospitals often provide the opportunity for people to watch their favorite television shows. Promoting routine activities can be taken to detrimental extremes, however. Nothing withers the spirit more than seeing a group of older adults listlessly lined up in chairs in a room in a nursing home watching endless hours of television.

I believe that far more could be done to capitalize on the familiar and everyday rituals. Here's an example. There are many places in the economically developing world where members of a patient's family come to the hospital, cook for, and even share a room with, the patient. This would hardly be tolerated in hospitals in the developed world, but the idea of having family nearby to care for a person is certainly a good one.

Providers *have* thought creatively about incorporating everyday routines and the familiar into health care settings. Recall the attempt to create a feeling of access to the outside world in Glasgow Homoeopathic Hospital, the focus of life around the kitchen at the Oakmont Alzheimer's facility, and the Web cam visits to residents in the Green House Project. The ideas are there; healing cultures need to be changed to embrace them.

Nattering Nabobs and Pollyanna Pundits

Throughout this book I have tried to persuade the reader of my conviction that there *are* specific steps that can be taken to improve environments in places that will be conducive to health. Too often, I feel, "critical" social scientists (and I count myself among this group) point out what is wrong with societal systems such as health care and stop there. Former U.S. vice president Spiro Agnew famously tried to belittle critical liberals as "nattering nabobs of negativism." Our function as criticizers hopefully is much more than that. There is no question that health care systems need to be shaken up. The abuses of those in power that Agnew and his ilk try to keep under wraps need to be exposed. But part of our responsibility, along with pointing out faults, is to suggest some strategies that will have beneficial effects. The danger, of course, is that we lean too far in the opposite direction and become "Pollyanna pundits of the positive," positive thinkers out to win friends and influence people by pretending that health care systems have no faults and that health providers are always doing the right thing.

I am well aware that my efforts to accentuate what has worked to achieve health environments in the past and present could be construed as wishful positive thinking. One could come away from this book with the impression that all one has to do is implement a specific design feature such as plant a garden in a hospital courtyard and all will be well. Of course that is not true. There is much more to healing than a garden. What works for one person does not for another. What I really seek to do is pursue a dialectic between extremes of unthinking optimism and demoralizing pessimism. Let us look for faults and correct them. Let us be creative and find acceptable ways to improve health. Let us implement design features and then evaluate them. Looking for specific aspects of natural, built, symbolic, and social environments that are conducive to health is one way to do this.

Conflicts and Their Resolution

In the conclusions to chapters 3 and 4, the idea that every potential healing place has inherent conflicts was raised. Not everyone agrees that places such as Bath and Lourdes are conducive to health. The nattering nabob dwells on these conflicts and might even go so far as to say that no place can be therapeutic. The Pollyanna pundit ignores the conflicts. I suggest steering a path between extremes, admitting that there are conflicts and trying to resolve them. Despite inherent conflicts, people are healed in many places.

I recently visited a state mental institution. I was given an extensive tour by the assistant director and also had a chance to talk with the chief building and grounds engineer and the director of the children's wing. I was happy to learn that staff had thought about my four environments, although they did not express their ideas in terms of that framework. As examples, some of the wallpaper in common areas in the children's wing showed natural scenes, and although bedrooms were austere they were also light and airy.

Although I was mostly given the point of view of senior administrative staff, the assistant director pointed out several issues that led to conflicts. A major problem arose because, although staff seemed to know about several specific design features that could be therapeutic, they could not afford them. In addition, they had to be extremely careful about implementing new ideas. For example, a picture of a natural scene such as a beach or a forest framed in glass and hung on a wall was out of the question as it could be used in a destructive way by a patient.

It became clear that the desire on the part of the staff to control patients could run counter to the ideas of organizations such as the Department of

Justice and human rights groups who monitored the hospital. Take the issue of restraining violent patients. Strait jackets were no longer used, but
beds in some rooms had leather straps attached to them for restraint. Were
these absolutely necessary? When should restraints of any kind be used? Is
sedating patients always a better alternative?

One particular focal point for potential conflict was the admitting
room. This place represents a boundary between the world outside the
institution and the world within. Typically, patients are admitted either
by family members or the police. They are often extremely angry and
even violent when they are taken into the admitting room. Hospital
staff, however, must by law be very careful not to strike patients or handle them roughly. In such a situation, the need to constrain conflicts
with the inclination of most providers to be humane. Issues of restraint
and conflicting modes of treatment are matters of continuing debate.
They need to be talked about. Ways need to be sought of resolving them
as they arise.

How to Do It

How does one actually go about creating a healing place? I suggest one
can think in terms of three processes: conceptualization, implementation,
and evaluation. In the conceptualization phase, the goal should be to create environments that are conducive to various types of healing, including physical, mental, emotional, and spiritual. As I hope this book has
shown, a focus on physical healing only is very limiting. Furthermore,
consideration of the different types of healing can lead to synergies that
increase the overall therapeutic atmosphere of a place.

The four environments elaborated throughout the book could be
used as a conceptual framework for thinking about specific design features. As we have seen, there are many examples of each type of environment to be considered. Indeed, there are almost too many ideas to
select from places such as Epidauros, Bath, and Lourdes, as well as from
the hospital design literature. These examples come immediately to
mind: breaking down status hierarchies (social environment), the concept of healing as a pilgrimage (symbolic environment), noise abate-
ment (built environment), and murals of natural scenes (natural environment). Planners have to decide which ideas are suitable in particular

situations. I suggest that, for the enterprise to be successful, conceptualization should be engaged in by a wide variety of actors: architects, administrators, staff, and patients.

Implementation, of course, is a process fraught with potential pitfalls. In the mental hospital visit mentioned above, the people I talked to had many good ideas about therapeutic design features but were constantly frustrated by the lack of funds to put them into place. So there are financial barriers to overcome. Then there is the problem of dealing with cultural inertia, of changing institutional cultures. Those involved in implementation must be flexible, constantly open to change and new ideas. Again, I believe that participation by many different groups of people is a key to success in implementation.

Evaluation is a notoriously neglected process. It is too easy to assume that once the thinking behind conceptualization and the doing behind implementation are over the design process is complete. But how well did specific design features really work to produce healing environments? Everyone involved should be asked about this, patients from different cultural, social, and economic backgrounds most of all. The four environments could be of value as an evaluative framework. A proper evaluation is bound to lead to many headaches, simply because those involved will have a wide range of perceptions about what is therapeutic and what is not. But conflicting perceptions must be dealt with and compromises made.

Works Cited

Anspach, Renee R. 1988. "Notes on the Sociology of Medical Discourse: The Language of Case Presentation." *Journal of Health and Social Behavior* 29: 357–75.

Anstey, Christopher. 1767. *The New Bath Guide: Or, Memoirs of the B-r-d Family*. 5th ed. London: J. Dodsley.

Austen-Leigh, Emma. 1939. *Jane Austen and Bath*. London: Spottiswoode, Ballantyne.

Ayensu, Edward S. 1981. "A Worldwide Role for the Healing Powers of Plants." *Smithsonian* 12: 86–97.

Bagley, C. 1974. "The Built Environment as an Influence on Personality and Social Behavior: A Spatial Study." Pp. 156–62 in *Psychology and the Built Environment*, edited by David Canter and Terence Lee. New York: John Wiley.

Bamborough, J. B. 1980. *The Little World of Man*. London: Longmans, Green.

Barbe, David. 1894. *Lourdes: Yesterday, Today, and Tomorrow*. London: Burns and Oates.

Bastien, Joseph W. 1985. "Qollahuaya-Andean Body Concepts: A Topographic-Hydraulic Model of Physiology." *American Anthropologist* 87: 595–611.

Bath and Bristol Guide: Or, The Tradesman's and Traveller's Pocket-Companion, The. 1755. Bath: T. Boddeley.

Beck, Alan M. 1986. "Use of Animals in the Rehabilitation of Psychiatric Patients." *Psychological Reports* 58: 63–66.

Becker, Franklin D. 1977. "The Effect of Physical Design Change on Organizational Changes and Behavior Patterns in a Hospital Nursing Unit." Pp. 105–62 in *User Participation, Personalization, and Environmental Meaning; Three Field Studies*. Program in Urban and Regional Studies. Ithaca, N.Y.: Cornell University.

Bell, Morag. 2001. "Comments on Therapeutic Landscape." Paper presented at Seminar 1: Wellbeing: The Interaction between Person and Environment. Economic and Social Research Council Seminar Series. Wellbeing: Social and Individual Determinants. St. Bartholomew's Hospital, London, September 11.

Bezzant, Norman. 1980. *Out of the Rock*. London: Heinemann.

Blumhagen, Dan W. 1979. "The Doctor's White Coat: The Image of the Physician in Modern America." *Annals of Internal Medicine* 91: 111–16.

Burford, Alison. 1969. *The Greek Temple Builders at Epidauros*. Toronto: University of Toronto Press.

Canter, Sandra, and David Canter. 1979. "Building for Therapy." Pp. 1–28 in *Designing for Therapeutic Environments*, edited by David Canter and Sandra Canter. New York: John Wiley & Sons.

Caton, Richard. 1900. *The Temples and Ritual of Asklepios at Epidauros and Athens*. 2nd ed. London: C. J. Clay and Sons.

Cayleff, Susan E. 1988. "Gender, Ideology, and the Water-Cure Movement." Pp. 82–98 in *Other Healers: Unorthodox Medicine in America*, edited by Norman Gevitz. Baltimore: Johns Hopkins University Press.

Chadwick, Audrey L. 1997. "The Healing Power of Gardens." Pp. 392–403 in *Reflections on Healing: A Central Nursing Construct*, edited by Phyllis Beck Kritek. New York: NLN Press.

Clark, Gordon L., and Michael Dear. 1984. "State Apparatus and Everyday Life." Pp. 60–82 in *State Apparatus and Everyday Life*, edited by Gordon L. Clark and Michael Dear. Boston: Allen & Unwin.

Coley, Noel G. 1982. "Physicians and the Chemical Analysis of Mineral Waters in Eighteenth-Century England." *Medical History* 26: 123–44.

———. 1990. "Physicians, Chemists and the Analysis of Mineral Waters: The Most Difficult Part of Chemistry." *Medical History* (Suppl. no. 10): 56–66.

Cornish, Claire V. 1997. "Behind the Crumbling Walls; The Re-Working of a Former Asylum's Geography." *Health & Place* 3, no. 3: 101–10.

Cranston, Ruth. 1955. *The Miracle of Lourdes*. New York: Doubleday.

Csordas, Thomas J. 1983. "The Rhetoric of Transformation in Ritual Healing." *Culture, Medicine, and Psychiatry* 7: 333–75.

Cunliffe, Barry. 1969. *Roman Bath*. Oxford: Oxford University Press.

———. 1986. *The City of Bath*. Gloucester: Alan Sutton.

Daniels, Stephen, and Denis Cosgrove. 1988. "Introduction: Iconography and Landscape." Pp. 1–10 in *The Iconography of Landscape*, edited by Denis Cosgrove and Stephen Daniels. Cambridge: Cambridge University Press.

Dobbs, G. Rebecca. 1997. "Interpreting the Navajo Sacred Geography as a Landscape of Healing." *Pennsylvania Geographer* 35, no. 2: 136–50.

Dow, James. 1986. "Universal Aspects of Symbolic Healing: A Theoretical Synthesis." *American Anthropologist* 88: 56–69.

Dubos, Rene. 1959. *Mirage of Health: Utopias, Progress, and Biological Change.* New York: Harper & Row.

Eade, John. 1992. "Pilgrimage and Tourism at Lourdes, France." *Annals of Tourism Research* 19, no. 1: 8–31.

Edelstein, Emma J., and Ludwig Edelstein. 1945. *Asclepius: A Collection and Interpretation of the Testimonies.* Vol. 2. Baltimore: Johns Hopkins University Press.

Edginton, Barry. 1997. "Moral Architecture: The Influence of the York Retreat on Asylum Design." *Health and Place* 3, no. 2: 91–99.

Eliade, Mircea. 1959. *The Sacred and the Profane: The Nature of Religion.* New York: Harcourt Brace Jovanovich.

Evans, Gary W. 1982. "General Introduction." Pp. 1–11 in *Environmental Stress,* edited by Gary W. Evans. Cambridge: Cambridge University Press.

Eyles, John, and Kevin J. Woods. 1983. *The Social Geography of Medicine and Health.* London: Croom Helm.

Fenton, Mary V. 1997. "Healing: The Outcome of Humanistic Care." Pp. 28–38 in *Reflections on Healing: A Central Nursing Construct,* edited by Phyllis Beck Kritek. New York: NLN Press.

Filstead, William J., and Jean J. Rossi. 1973. "Therapeutic Milieu, Therapeutic Community, and Milieu Therapy: Some Conceptual and Definitional Distinctions." Pp. 3–13 in *The Therapeutic Community: A Sourcebook of Readings,* edited by Jean J. Rossi and William J. Filstead. New York: Behavioral Publishers.

Flarey, Dominick L. 1991. "The Social Climate Scale: A Tool for Organizational Change and Development." *Journal of Nursing Administration* 21, no. 4: 37–44.

Fox, Nicholas J. 1993. *Postmodernism, Sociology and Health.* Buckingham: Open University Press.

Frank, Jerome D., and Julia Frank. 1991. *Persuasion and Healing: A Comparative Study of Psychotherapy.* Baltimore: Johns Hopkins University Press.

Frazer, James George. 1898. *Pausanius's Description of Greece: Translated with a Commentary.* London: Macmillan.

Frede, Michael. 1987. *Philosophy and Medicine in Antiquity. Essays in Ancient Philosophy.* Minneapolis: University of Minnesota Press.

Gadd, David. 1971. *Georgian Summer: Bath in the Eighteenth Century.* Bath: Adams and Dart.

Gerlach-Spriggs, Nancy, Richard Enoch Kaufman, and Sam Bass Warner Jr. 1998. *Restorative Gardens: The Healing Landscape.* New Haven, Conn.: Yale University Press.

Gesler, Wilbert M. 1992. "Therapeutic Landscapes: Medical Geographic Research in Light of the New Cultural Geography." *Social Science and Medicine* 34, no. 7: 735–46.

———. 1993. "Therapeutic Landscapes: Theory and a Case Study of Epidauros, Greece." *Environment and Planning D: Society and Space* 11: 171–89.

———. 1996. "Lourdes: Healing in a Place of Pilgrimage." *Health and Place* 2, no. 2: 95–105.

———. 1998. "Bath's Reputation as a Healing Place." Pp. 17–35 in *Putting Health into Place*, edited by R. A. Kearns and W. M. Gesler. Syracuse: Syracuse University Press.

Gesler, Wilbert M., Morag Bell, and Sarah E. Curtis. 2002. "Therapeutic Environments and the Hospital Design Process: A Critique." Unpublished paper.

Gevitz, Norman. 1988. "Osteopathic Medicine: From Deviance to Difference." Pp. 124–56 in *Other Healers: Unorthodox Medicine in America*, edited by Norman Gevitz. Baltimore: Johns Hopkins University Press.

Gibbons, Flachra. 2001. "Hospitals Wary at Offer of Hirst's Body Parts Art." *Guardian* (December 3): 9.

Gifford, Blair D., and Ross M. Mullner. 1988. "Modeling Hospital Closure Relative to Organizational Theory: The Application of Ecology Theory's Environmental Determinism and Adaptation Perspectives." *Social Science and Medicine* 27, no. 11: 1287–94.

Gladwell, Malcolm. 1997. "The Alzheimer's Strain: How to Accommodate Too Many Patients." *New Yorker* (October 20–27): 125–29.

———. 2000. *The Tipping Point: How Little Things Can Make a Big Difference*. London: Little, Brown.

Godkin, Michael A. 1980. "Identity and Place: Clinical Application Based on Notions of Rootedness and Uprootedness." Pp. 73–85 in *The Human Experience of Space and Place*, edited by Anne Buttimer and David Seamon. Andover, Hants.: Croom Helm.

Gold, Mick. 1985. "A History of Nature." Pp. 12–33 in *Geography Matters!* edited by D. Massey and J. Allen. Cambridge: Cambridge University Press.

Good, Byron J. 1994. *Medicine, Rationality, and Experience: An Anthropological Perspective*. Cambridge: Cambridge University Press.

Gordon, Rena, Barbara Nienstedt, and Wilbert M. Gesler, eds. 1998. *Alternative Therapies: Expanding Options in Health Care*. New York: Springer.

Green House Project. 2002. "The Idea. Rationale." The Green House Project, 2002. Available at thegreenhouseproject.com/idea.htm.

Griffin, Joyce P. 1992. "The Impact of Noise on Critically Ill People." *Holistic Nurse Practitioner* 6, no. 4: 53–56.

Habicht, Christian. 1985. *Pausanius' Guide to Ancient Greece*. Berkeley: University of California Press.

Haddon, John. 1973. *Bath*. London: B. T. Batsford.

Hagey, Rebecca. 1984. "The Phenomenon, the Explanations and the Responses: Metaphors Surrounding Diabetes in Urban Canadian Indians." *Social Science and Medicine* 18: 265–72.

Hamilton, Mary. 1906. *Incubation or the Cure of Disease in Pagan Temples and Christian Churches*. London: W. C. Henderson & Son.

Hamlin, Christopher. 1990. "Chemistry, Medicine, and the Legitimization of English Spas, 1740–1840." *Medical History* (Suppl. no. 10): 67–81.

Harley, David. 1990. "A Sword in a Madman's Hand: Professional Opposition to Popular Consumption in the Waters Literature of Southern England and the Midlands, 1570–1870." *Medical History* (Suppl. no. 10): 48–55.

Helman, Cecil G. 1994. *Culture, Health, and Illness*. 3rd ed. Oxford: Butterworth-Heineman.

Holahan, Charles J. 1979. "Environmental Psychology in Psychiatric Hospital Settings." Pp. 213–31 in *Designing for Therapeutic Environments*, edited by David Canter and Sandra Canter. New York: John Wiley & Sons.

Howard, J., F. David, C. Pope, and S. Ruzek. 1977. "Humanizing Health Care: The Implications of Technology, Centralizing, and Self-Care." *Medical Care* 5 (Suppl. no. 15): 11–26.

Hunter, John M. 1973. "Geophagy in Africa and the United States: A Culture-Nutrition Hypothesis." *Geographical Review* 63: 170–95.

Hunter, John M., Oscar H. Horst, and Robert N. Thomas. 1989. "Religious Geophagy as a Cottage Industry: The Holy Clay Tablets of Esquipulas, Guatemala." *National Geographic Research* 5, no. 3: 281–95.

Hutton, James D., and Lynne D. Richardson. 1995. "Healthscapes: The Role of Facility and Physical Environment on Consumer Attitudes, Satisfaction, Quality Assessments, and Behaviors." *Health Care Management Review* 20, no. 2: 48–61.

Illich, Ivan. 1976. *Medical Nemesis: The Expropriation of Health*. New York: Pantheon Books.

Improved Bath Guide, The. 1825. London: S. Simms.

Jackson, Peter. 1989. *Maps of Meaning: An Introduction to Cultural Geography*. London: Unwin Hyman.

Jackson, Ralph. 1990. "Waters and Spas in the Classical World." *Medical History* (Suppl. no. 10): 1–13.

Janzen, John M. 1978. "The Comparative Study of Medical Systems as Changing Social Systems." *Social Science and Medicine* 12: 121–29.

Jones, Maxwell. 1979. "The Therapeutic Community, Social Learning and Social Change." Pp. 1–9 in *Therapeutic Communities: Reflections and Progress*, edited by R. D. Henshelwood and Nick Manning. London: Routledge & Kegan
Paul.

Katz, Pearl. 1981. "Ritual in the Operating Room." *Ethnology* 20: 335–50.

Kearns, Robin A. 1991. "The Place of Health in the Health of Place: The Case
of the Hokianga Special Medical Area." *Social Science and Medicine* 33:
519–30.

Kearns, Robin A., and Wilbert M. Gesler, eds. 1998. *Putting Health into Place:
Landscape, Identity, and Well-Being*. Syracuse: Syracuse University Press.

Kearns, Robin A., and J. Ross Barnett. 1997. "Consumerist Ideology and the
Symbolic Landscapes of Private Medicine." *Health and Place* 3: 171–80.

———. 1999. "To Boldly Go? Place Metaphor and the Marketing of Auckland's
Starship Hospital." *Environment and Planning D: Society and Space* 17: 201–26.

Kellert, Stephen R., and Edward O. Wilson, eds. 1993. *The Biophilia Hypothesis*.
Washington, D.C.: Island Press.

Kenny, Cheryl, and David Canter. 1979. "Evaluating Acute General Hospitals."
Pp. 309–32 in *Designing for Therapeutic Environments*, edited by D. Canter and
S. Canter. New York: John Wiley & Sons.

Kerenyi, Karl. 1960. *Asklepios: Archetypal Image of the Physician's Existence*. London: Thames and Hudson.

Kleinman, Arthur. 1973. "Medicine's Symbolic Reality: On a Central Problem
in the Philosophy of Medicine." *Inquiry* 16: 206–13.

———. 1978. "Concepts and a Model for the Comparison of Medical Systems as
Cultural Systems." *Social Science and Medicine* 12: 85–93.

———. 1988. *The Illness Narratives: Suffering, Healing, and the Human Condition*.
New York: Basic Books.

Krause, Elliott A. 1977. "The Historical Context of Health." Pp. 9–30 in *Power
and Illness: The Political Sociology of Health and Medical Care*. New York: Else-
vier.

Kritek, Phyllis Beck. 1997. "Healing: A Central Nursing Construct-Reflections
on Meaning." Pp. 11–27 in *Reflections on Healing: A Central Nursing Construct*,
edited by Phyllis Beck Kritek. New York: NLN Press.

Laderman, Carol. 1987. "The Ambiguity of Symbols in the Structure of Healing." *Social Science and Medicine* 24, no. 4: 293–301.

Landis, B. J. 1997. "Healing and the Human Spirit." Pp. 72–80 in *Reflections on
Healing: A Central Nursing Construct*, edited by Phyllis Beck Kritek. New York:
NLN Press.

Lawrence, Elizabeth Atwood. 1993. "The Sacred Bee, the Filthy Pig, and the Bat
out of Hell: Animal Symbolism as Cognitive Biophilia." Pp. 301–41 in *The*

Biophilia Hypothesis, edited by S. R. Kellert and E. O. Wilson. Washington, D.C.: Island Press.

Leatt, Peggy, and Rodney Schneck. 1982. "Work Environments in Different Types of Nursing Subunits." *Journal of Advanced Nursing* 7: 581–94.

Lees-Milne, James, and David Ford. 1982. *Images of Bath*. Richmond-Upon-Thames: Saint Helena Press.

Ley, David. 1981. "Behavioral Geography and the Philosophies of Meaning." Pp. 209–30 in *Behavioral Problems in Geography Revisited*, edited by Kevin R. Cox and Reginald C. Golledge. New York: Methuen.

Lown, Bernard. 1983. "Introduction." Pp. 11–28 in *The Healing Heart*, edited by Norman Cousins. New York: W. W. Norton.

Lloyd, Geoffrey Ernest Richard. 1979. *Magic, Reason, and Experience: Studies in the Origin and Development of Greek Science*. Cambridge: Cambridge University Press.

———, ed. 1983. *Hippocratic Writings*. London: Penguin Books.

Macdonald, M. R., J. J. Schentag, W. B. Ackerman, and R. Walsh. 1981. "ICU Nurses Rate Their Work Places." *Hospitals* 55, no. 2: 115–16, 188.

Macmon. 2001. *Glasgow Homoeopathic Hospital*. Glasgow: Maclachlan Monaghan.

Manning, Nick P. 1989. *The Therapeutic Community Movement: Charisma and Routinization*. New York: Routledge.

Marnham, Patrick. 1980. *Lourdes: A Modern Pilgrimage*. London: Heinemann.

Marx, Leo. 1968. "Pastoral Ideals and City Troubles." Pp. 119–44 in *The Fitness of Man's Environment*. Washington, D.C.: Smithsonian Institution Press.

McIntyre, Sylvia. 1981. "Bath: The Rise of a Resort Town, 1660–1800." Pp. 198–247 in *Country Towns in Pre-industrial England*, edited by Peter Clark. New York: St. Martin's Press.

Mehl, L. E. 1986. *Mind and Matter: A Healing Approach to Chronic Illness*. Berkeley, Calif.: Mindbody Press.

Meier, Carl Alfred. 1967. *Ancient Incubation and Modern Psychotherapy*. Evanston, Ill.: Northwestern University Press.

Meinig, Donald William. 1979. "Introduction." Pp. 1–7 in *The Interpretation of Ordinary Landscapes*, edited by Donald William Meinig. New York: Oxford University Press.

Meyer, Judith W., and Ellen K. Cromley. 1989. "Caregiving Environments and Elderly Residential Mobility." *Professional Geographer* 41: 440–50.

Miles, Malcolm. 1997. "Art in Health Services." Pp. 150–63 in *Art, Space, and the City: Public Art and Urban Futures*. London: Routledge.

Mills, William J. 1982. "Metaphorical Vision: Changes in Western Attitudes to the Environment." *Annals of the Association of American Geographers* 66: 309–22.

Minckley, Barbara Blake. 1968. "A Study of Noise and its Relationship to Patient Discomfort in the Recovery Room." *Nursing Research* 17, no. 3: 247–50.

Mishler, Elliott G. 1984. *The Discourse of Medicine: Dialectics of Medical Interviews*. Norwood, N.J.: Ablex Publishing.

Mitchell, Bridgette. 1986. "English Spas." Pp. 189–204 in *Bath History*, Vol. I. Oxford: Alan Sutton.

Moos, Rudolf H. 1977a. "Understanding Treatment Programs and Outcomes." Pp. 1–19 in *Evaluating Treatment Environments: The Quality of Psychiatric and Substance Abuse Programs*, edited by Rudolf H. Moos. 2nd ed. New Brunswick, N.J.: Transaction Publishers.

———. 1977b. "The Social Climate of Hospital Programs." Pp. 23–44 in *Evaluating Treatment Environments: The Quality of Psychiatric and Substance Abuse Programs*, edited by Rudolf H. Moos. 2nd ed. New Brunswick, N.J.: Transaction Publishers.

Morrice, J. K. W. 1979. "Basic Concepts: A Critical Review." Pp. 49–58 in *Therapeutic Communities: Reflection and Progress*, edited by R. D. Hinshelwood and Nick Manning. London: Routledge & Kegan Paul.

Moss, Nancy. 1984. "Hospital Units as Social Contexts: Effects on Natural Behavior." *Social Science and Medicine* 19, no. 5: 515–22.

Moyers, Bill. 1993. *Healing and the Mind*. New York: Doubleday.

Navarro, Vicente. 1974. "The Underdevelopment of Health or the Health of Underdevelopment: An Analysis of the Distribution of Human Health Resources in Latin America." *International Journal of Health Services* 4: 5–27.

Neale, Ron. 1973a. "Society, Belief, and the Building of Bath, 1700–1793." Pp. 253–80 in *Landscape and Society*, edited by Christopher W. Chalkin and M. Havinden. London: Longman.

———. 1973b. "Bath: Ideology and Utopia, 1700–1760." *Studies in the Eighteenth Century* 3: 37–54.

Neame, Alan. 1968. *The Happening at Lourdes*. London: Hodder and Stoughton.

Neve, Michael Raymond. 1984. "Natural Philosophy, Medicine and the Culture of Science in Provincial England: The Cases of Bristol, 1790–1850, and Bath, 1750–1820." Ph.D. diss., University College, London.

Nightingale, Florence. 1863. *Notes on Hospitals*. 3rd ed. London: Longman, Green, Longman, Roberts, and Green.

Nolan, Mary Lee, and Sidney Nolan. 1989. *Christian Pilgrimage in Modern Western Europe*. Chapel Hill: University of North Carolina Press.

Nouwen, Henri J. M. 1990. "A Sudden Trip to Lourdes." *New Oxford Review* 57: 7–13.

Nuffield Provincial Hospitals Trust. 1955. *Studies in the Functions and Design of Hospitals*. London: Oxford University Press.

Nutton, Vivian. 1985. "Murders and Miracles: Lay Attitudes towards Medicine in Classical Antiquity." Pp. 25–53 in *Patients and Practitioners: Lay Perceptions in Pre-industrial Society*, edited by Roy Porter. Cambridge: Cambridge University Press.

Paignon, Echon. 1956. "A Marian Meditation." *America* 95: 62, 164.

Papastamou, Dimitrios. 1977. *Asklipios-Epidauros and Their Museum*. Athens: Apollo Editions.

Parker, Robert. 1983. *Miasma: Pollution and Purification in Early Greek Religion*. Oxford: Clarendon Press.

Pausanius. 1971. *Guide to Greece* Volume 1: *Central Greece*. London: Penguin Books.

Philo, Chris. 1987. "Fit Locations for an Asylum: The Historical Geography of the Nineteenth Century 'Mad-Business' in England as Viewed through the Pages of the *Asylum Journal*." *Journal of Historical Geography* 13: 398–415.

Plotkin, Mark J. 1993. *Tales of a Shaman's Apprentice*. New York: Penguin.

Pope, Barbara Cornado. 1989. "Emile Zola's Lourdes: Land of Healing and Rapture." *Literature and Medicine* 8: 22–35.

Porter, Rose, and Phyllis Watson. 1985. "Environment: The Healing Difference." *Nursing Management* 16, no. 6: 19–24.

Porter, Roy. 1990. "Introduction, The Medical History of Waters and Spas." *Medical History* (Suppl. no. 10): vii–xii.

Pred, Alan. 1983. "Structuration and Place: On the Becoming of Sense of Place and Structure of Feeling." *Journal for the Theory of Social Behavior* 13: 45–68.

Price, Laurie. 1987. "Ecuadorian Illness Stories: Cultural Knowledge in Natural Discourse." Pp. 313–42 in *Cultural Models in Language and Thought*, edited by Dorothy Holland and Naomi Quinn. Cambridge: Cambridge University Press.

Purvis, Andrew. 2001. "Is It a Hotel? Is It a Trendy Car? No, It's a Hospital." *Guardian* (August 5): 14.

Quinn, Janet F. 1997. "Foreword." Pp. vii–x in *Reflections on Healing: A Central Nursing Construct*, edited by Phyllis Beck Kritek. New York: NLN Press.

Rahtz, Philip, and Lorna Watts. 1986. "The Archaeologist on the Road to Lourdes and Santiago de Compostela." Pp. 51–73 in *The Anglo Saxon Church*, edited by Lawrence A. S. Butler and Richard K. Morris. London: Council for British Archaeology.

Ranger, Terence. 1982. "Introduction." Pp. xi–xxiv in *The Church and Healing*, edited by W. J. Shields. Oxford: Basil Blackwell.

Rees, Kevin. 1985. "Medicine as a Commodity: Hydrotherapy in Matlock." *Society for the Social History of Medicine Bulletin* 36: 24–27.

Reizenstein, Janet E. 1982. "Hospital Design and Human Behavior: A Review of the Recent Literature." Pp. 137–69 in *Advances in Environmental Psychology*, Volume 4, *Environment and Health*. Hillsdale, N.J.: Lawrence Erlbaum Associates.

Report of the Bath Society for the Suppression of Vagrants. Bath: Bath Society, 1810.

Rinschede, Gisbert. 1986–87."The Pilgrimage Town of Lourdes." *Journal of Cultural Geography* 7: 21–34.

Rolls, Roger. 1978. "In Pursuit of the Cure." Pp. 47–50 in *Bath-Museum City?* edited by G. Hanes. Bath: Bath University Press.

———. 1988. *The Hospital of the Nation*. Bath: Bird Publications.

Rosengren, William R., and Spencer DeVault. 1963. "The Sociology of Time and Space in an Obstetrical Hospital." Pp. 266–92 in *The Hospital in Modern Society*, edited by Eliot Friedson. New York: Free Press of Glencoe.

Rossi, Ernest L. 1986. *The Psychobiology of Mind-Body Healing*. New York: W. W. Norton.

Rowntree, Lester B., and Margaret W. Conkey. 1980. "Symbolism and the Cultural Landscape." *Annals of the Association of American Geographers* 70: 459–74.

Russell, James A., and Lawrence M. Ward. 1982. "Environmental Psychology." *Annual Review of Psychology* 33: 651–88.

Ryden, Muriel B. 1985. "Environmental Support for Autonomy in the Institutionalized Elderly." *Research in Nursing and Health* 8: 363–71.

Schama, Simon. 1988. *The Embarrassment of Riches: An Interpretation of Dutch Culture in the Golden Age*. New York: Fontana Press.

Schnorrenberg, Barbara Brandon. 1984. "Medical Men of Bath." *Studies in Eighteenth Century Culture* 13: 189–203.

Scott, Lisa. 1992. "Treatment Centers a Laboratory for Facility Design." *Modern Healthcare* (December 7): 30, 32.

———. 2002. Presbyterian SeniorCare, Oakmont, PA. Personal Communication.

Scully, Vincent. 1969. *The Earth, the Temple, and the Gods: Greek Sacred Architecture*. Rev. ed. New York: Frederick A. Praeger.

Singh, J. 1990. "A Multifacet Typology of Patient Satisfaction with a Hospital Stay." *Journal of Health Care Marketing* 10: 8–21.

Sitwell, Edith. 1987. *Bath*. London: Faber & Faber.

Spencer, Christopher, and Mark Blades. 1986. "Pattern and Process: An Essay on the Relationship between Behavioral Geography and Environmental Psychology." *Progress in Human Geography* 10: 230–48.

Staiano, Kathryn Vance. 1979. "A Semiotic Definition of Illness." *Semiotica* 28: 107–25.

Stam, Henderikus J., and Nicholas P. Spanos. 1982. "The Asclepian Dream Healings and Hypnosis: A Critique." *International Journal of Clinical and Experimental Hypnosis* 30, no. 1: 9–22.

Stewart, Bob. 1981. *The Waters of the Gap: The Mythology of Aquae Sulis*. Bath: Bath City Council.

Stokols, Daniel. 1978. "Environmental Psychology." *Annual Review of Psychology* 29: 253–95.

Struckmann, Reinhard. 1979. *Important Medical Centres in Antiquity: Epidauros and Corinth.* Athens: Editions Kasas.

Sumption, Jonathan. 1975. *Pilgrimage: An Image of Medieval Religion.* New York: Faber & Faber.

Tambiah, S. J. 1968. "The Magical Power of Words." *Man* 3, no. 2: 175–208.

Thomas, Keith. 1971. *Religion and the Decline of Magic: Studies in Popular Beliefs in Sixteenth and Seventeenth Century England.* London: Penguin Books.

Todd, Alexandra Dundas, and Sue Fisher. 1993. *The Social Organization of Doctor-Patient Communication.* 2nd ed. Norwood, N.J.: Ablex Publishing.

Tomlinson, Richard Allan. 1983. *Epidauros.* London: Granada.

Tuan, Yi-Fu. 1974. "Space and Place: Humanistic Perspective." *Progress in Geography* 6: 211–52.

Turner, Victor, and Edith Turner. 1978. *Image and Pilgrimage in Christian Culture.* Oxford: Basil Blackwell.

Ulrich, Roger S. 1984. "View through a Window May Influence Recovery from Surgery." *Science* 224: 420–21.

Ulrich, Roger S., Robert F. Simons, Barbara D. Losito, Evelyn Fiorito, Mark A. Miles, and Michael Zelson. 1991. "Stress Recovery during Exposure to Natural and Urban Environments." *Journal of Environmental Psychology* 11: 201–30.

Vance, James E., Jr. 1972. "California and the Search for the Ideal." *Annals of the Association of American Geographers* 62: 185–210.

Verderber, Stephen. 1986. "Dimensions of Person-Window Transactions in the Hospital Environment." *Environment and Behavior* 18, no. 4: 450–66.

Walter, Eugene Victor. 1988. *Placeways: A Theory of the Human Environment.* Chapel Hill: University of North Carolina Press.

Williams, Allison, ed. 1999. *Therapeutic Landscapes: The Dynamic between Place and Wellness.* Lanham, Md.: University Press of America.

Williams, Margaret A. 1988. "The Physical Environment and Patient Care." *Annual Review of Nursing Research* 6: 61–84.

Williams, Raymond. 1973. *The Country and the City.* New York: Oxford University Press.

Wilson, Larkin M. 1972. "Intensive Care Delirium: The Effect of Outside Deprivation in a Windowless Unit." *Archives of Internal Medicine* 130: 225–26.

Winsor, Diana. 1980. *The Dream of Bath.* Bath: Travel & Trade Publications.

Wood, John. 1765. *An Essay towards a Description of Bath.* London.

Wordsworth, William. 1975. *Selected Poems,* edited by Walford Davies. London: J. M. Dent and Sons.

Wriston, Barbara. 1978. *Rare Doings at Bath*. Chicago: Art Institute of Chicago.

Zimdars-Swartz, Sandra. 1991. *Encountering Mary: From LaSalette to Medjugorje*. Princeton, N.J.: Princeton University Press.

Zola, Irving Kenneth. 1972. "Medicine As an Institution of Social Control." *Sociological Review* 20: 487–504.

Index

About the Author

Professor **Wilbert Gesler** received his Ph.D. in geography from the University of North Carolina at Chapel Hill in 1978. He also has M.A. degrees in mathematics (The Pennsylvania State University) and English literature (Indiana University of Pennsylvania). His principal teaching and research interests are in health geography and cultural geography. Among his publications are *The Cultural Geography of Health Care* (University of Pittsburgh Press) and, with Dr. Robin A. Kearns, *Culture/Place/Health* (Routledge).